Role of Sustainability Impact Assessment in Public Health Policy Change

Francis Sarr

CENMEDRA

Published by CENMEDRA – the Centre for Media and Development Research in Africa

First published in The Gambia by Bohnjack Group Limited in 2013

This edition published by CENMEDRA in 2018

www.cenmedra.org

ISBN: 978-9983-960-19-8

Front cover design by Sadibou Kamaso

Layout design by Folashade Lasisi

www.cenmedra.org

info@cenmedra.org

Contents

List of Figures, Tables and Boxes

Figures:

Tables:

Boxes:

Dedication

This book is dedicated to the entire family of Sangol and Tedene Sarr (my parents), particularly my late brother Moses Latirr Sarr who also loved writing, though in a field different from health – agricultural education – a subject he knew so well and was so passionate about, and liked to discuss with anyone who had the time and patience to listen to him.

About the author

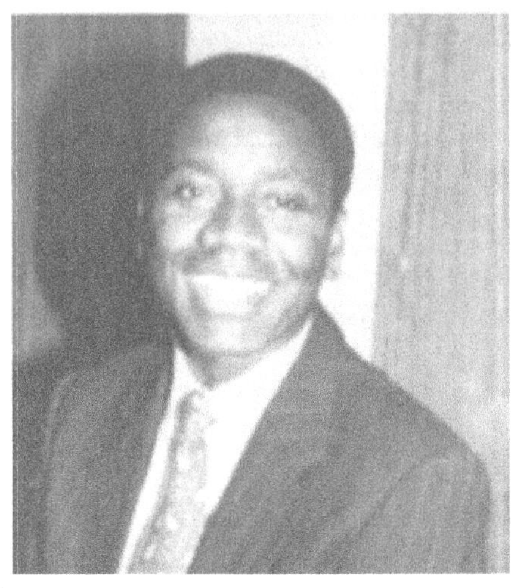

Francis Sarr, Associate Professor of Community Health Education and Fellow of the West African College of Nursing, is the Dean of the School of Graduate Studies and Research of the University of The Gambia. He was educated at The Gambia School of Nursing and Midwifery (SRN Cert.); Pharmacy Department at The Gambia's Ministry of Health (Medical Aide Cert.); Cuttington University College, Liberia (BSc Nursing); University of Wales, Cardiff (M Ed, Curriculum Development & Educational Administration); London University School of Hygiene and Tropical Medicine (MSc & Postgraduate Diploma, Public Health); London University Institute of Child Health (Nutrition & Child Health Cert.); and London South Bank University (PhD, Public Health).

He has a career in the health service that spans over a decade of working as a staff nurse and dispenser in urban and rural health services and 33 years of teaching in nursing and midwifery education. He participated in the planning of Primary Health Care (PHC) in The Gambia at headquarters and lower levels and was instrumental in the orientation of nursing and midwifery programmes to the PHC approach. A dedicated public health scholar and practitioner, Sarr is passionate about innovative approaches to healthcare education in the global South.

About CENMEDRA

CENMEDRA – the Centre for Media and Development Research in Africa – is a knowledge centre. Registered as an educational charity in The Gambia on 3 March 2014 it aims to promote, facilitate and disseminate research in media, communication and development in Africa. Its activities are focused on five main areas namely media research, researching development, new media and society, education, and publication. In line with its underlying aim of research application, it shares its research results with policymakers, media and development practitioners, media houses, regulators, scholars, politicians, librarians, activists, donors, development agencies, and the wider research community. It has a two-tiered governance structure: a board of trustees drawn from the media, civil society and academia, which provides strategy and policy direction, and an administrative secretariat that is responsible for operations and policy implementation.

MISSION

CENMEDRA exists to foster innovative research that puts Africa on the path of peace, progress and prosperity.

VISION

CENMEDRA envisions an enlightened African society, free from the burden of ignorance, where everyone is able to realise their fullest potential in peace and prosperity.

VALUES

- Integrity
- Openness
- Creativity
- Diligence

"There is only one good – knowledge, and one evil – ignorance."
Socrates (circa 470-399BC)

http://www.cenmedra.org
Email: info@cenmedra.org

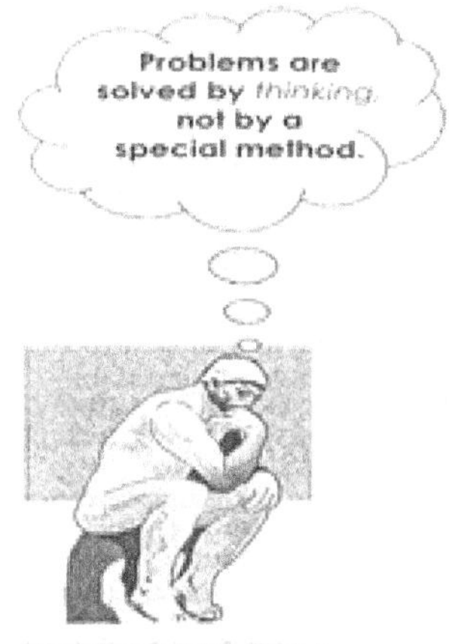

Preface

Much of what has been written about public health gives global attention to the burden of disease and the health implications of policies that are put in place to prevent disease and promote health. This is because significant improvements in the health of people globally can only be realized if attention is given to the root causes of ill health and to the policies and programmes that are designed to address them. The entire world population shares many of the established causes of disease. Each year, millions of people die of preventable deaths. For example, in 2012 non-communicable diseases caused 68% of all deaths globally, an increase from 60% in 2000. Cardiovascular diseases, cancer, diabetes and chronic lung diseases are four major non-communicable diseases. In the same period, communicable diseases (e.g. malaria) maternal (e.g. post-partum hemorrhage), neonatal (e.g. birth asphyxia) and nutrition (e.g. anemia) conditions were together chargeable for 23% of global deaths. Injuries were responsible for 9% of all deaths (WHO 2015). Thus, policies that deal with such causes of ill health can have wide effects on the public generally, as well as high-risk population groups.

But societies often do not understand the health implications of the various policies, strategies and programmes that societies normally formulate and implement. Notwithstanding, these decisions and actions could significantly impact the health of the population and health disparities. The health consequences can have economic and social costs, which can have multiplying and cumulative effects, such as the obesity epidemic in many countries related to the mass production and distribution of energy-dense foods. Identifying the potential effects in advance is fundamental for disease prevention and could have important consequences for trends in diseases and for social inequalities in a wide variety of health outcomes (National Academy of Sciences, 2011).

The importance of policy change to public health rests, firstly, on the recognition that the development of healthy public policy is a foundation of the new public health (WHO 1986). Secondly, public health programmes are developed to represent the policy goals of local health systems. Despite this recognition health effects may not be systematically included into decisions regarding policies, programmes, etc (National Academy of Sciences, 2011). Health research and the translation of findings to action is critical to making this transition and improving public health policy.

Impact assessment is concerned with assessing the positive and negative effects of potential and existing interventions at the policy level. The aim of impact assessment is to improve the evidence base on which decisions are made, and thereby improve the quality of decision-making. In the public health sector, impact assessment can be used by policymakers as a means of informing public policy and rule setting choices. Public regulation, whether in the form of policy or rules, can be good or bad, and it is unlikely, therefore, that the case for or against a regulatory measure can be convincingly made from first principles or on an a priori basis. An underlying rationale for impact assessment, therefore, is that public interventions need to be assessed on a case by case basis (Kirkpatrick et al, 2001).

The development of a methodology for assessing the impact of policy or rules is still at a formative stage, and the use of such methods in public decision-making is only beginning to gain acceptance (Kirkpatrick et al, 2001). The case for applying impact assessment at the project level is well established, and the methods of economic impact assessment (cost-benefit analysis) and environmental impact assessment, for example, are widely known. However, the development of a methodology for impact assessment at the strategic level (policy, plans and programmes) is at a much earlier stage (Kirkpatrick et al, 2001). At this level, impact assessment is given many names, including strategic impact assessment, regulatory impact assessment, integrated impact assessment, and sustainability impact assessment (e.g. OECD 2010; Kirkpatrick et al, 2001), which is the subject of this book..

Sustainability Impact Assessment (SIA) can be defined as a methodology for identifying and assessing the likelihood and scale of the economic, social and environmental impacts of intervention, in the form of a policy change or rules-measure (EU 2003). It emphasizes the importance of internalizing the principles of sustainable development into the development of all strategies from the beginning, and is aimed at being an integral part of the process of developing any strategy. The purpose is to ensure that those charged with making policy have the most complete information possible to guide them in their decision-making. To this end, SIA should include processes of consultation and participation with stakeholders and other interested parties (WHO 2001). Accordingly, SIA has been used since 1999 to advance international, EU and national governance by guaranteeing greater coherence of EU policies, giving an overview of problems, guaranteeing greater reliability through transparency and consultation and guaranteeing openness of the policy-making process through linking stakeholders and developing countries with EU policy analysis (EC 2003).

The UK government's position regarding sustainable development is, for example, set out in the UK Strategy for Sustainable Development "A Better Quality of Life" and states that local authorities should assess the sustainability implications of their development plan policies through sustainability appraisal. This is quite logical in transparent systems, and good planning systems inevitably look at social, economic and environmental aspects of the plans (WHO, 2001). Despite its importance in the development of public health policy, however, Sustainability Impact Assessment or appraisal lags behind other forms of impact assessments, such as Sustainability Environmental Assessment (SEA) and it is institutionalized in very few jurisdictions because there is, among other things, a lack of political will to introduce it in many cases (OECD, 2010). The only institutionalization of sustainable impact assessment is "Sustainability Appraisal" in the UK which is applied to land use and regional development planning; however, it is not mandatory and seemingly excludes health effects (OECD, 2010). Some reasons why health effects may not be systematically included into decisions regarding policies, programmes, projects, or plans in the US, for example, are the failure to capture health impacts adequately in the context of environmental impact assessments; structural and administrative barriers to collaboration among public-health, planning and environmental-health professionals; lack of a mandate or funding to assess the health impacts of planned policies and decisions; the perception that health and health disparities are attributable only to individual characteristics and choices; and the lack of inclusive and participatory mechanisms and processes for systematically integrating planning, public health, and environmental-health promotion in decision-making (National Academy of Sciences, 2011). Systematic processes for rigorously assessing health impacts are required. Though many deliberative and analytical tools are currently employed to include components of health into decisions, none of the tools completely gives all the needed characteristics (National Academy of Sciences, 2011).

The aim of this book is to present a methodological approach for assessing the sustainability of immunization programmes that illustrates the role Sustainability Impact Assessment can play in the assessment of public health policy change processes. The framework is based upon the premise that public health policy development issues should be addressed within an analysis of policy change that considers involvement and participation of stakeholders in assessment of policy change in a much broader way. Progress in developing meaningful health policy will require accepting the validity of stakeholder participation and developing frameworks that see stakeholders working together to develop and achieve public health goals. The methodological approach and framework is contingent on a case study related to immunization policy in The Gambia that focused on developing appropriate tools and assessing EPI sustainability, institutional and behavioural factors which affect the efficiency and sustainability of the EPI services and policy for improving or maintaining the level of immunization services.

Francis Sarr

Structure of the book

This book is divided into eleven chapters. Chapters 1, 2 and 3 present analyses of the concepts of public health, sustainability and policy change. Chapters 4 and 5 describe the stakeholder analysis and national health accounts frameworks. These chapters determine the attributes, characteristics and other features of these concepts and frameworks. The aim is to improve general clarity and understanding of these concepts and frameworks that contribute to the Sustainability Impact Assessment framework and the case study methodological approach that exemplifies its role in sustainability assessment of policy change in immunization systems. Chapter 6 outlines the Sustainability Impact Assessment framework itself, setting out the steps involved in a typical SIA with examples of methodologies used in the case study. Chapter 7 describes the case study methodological approach including its rationale and components. Chapter 8 outlines the application context of the case study with emphasis on the country's immunization system. Chapters 9 and 10 describe the application scenarios of the methodological approach, detailing the stakeholder analysis and resource map assessment processes. The summary and conclusions of the book are provided in Chapter 11. This chapter reviews the contributions of the Sustainability Impact Assessment framework and case study methodological approach, providing additional discussion of relevant issues and some directions for future work.

1

Public Health

The world has witnessed over the past century significant improvements in the health of populations. The rate of such change has increased rapidly in low -and middle –income countries following the Bretton Woods Conference in July 1944 (at which the International Monetary Fund and the World Bank were created). As will be seen in this chapter, public health has advanced these betterments to a degree that far outweighs the benefits of medical care. But such improvements have not been realized by all peoples of the world, as shown by the relatively higher burden of disease in developing countries when compared to developed countries. This chapter defines public health, gives a brief history of the field, and summarizes its many features including its functions, achievements and challenges. The chapter also outlines the implications for research and public health practice. The aim of this chapter is to describe public health as the context within which to situate in following chapters the analyses of other concepts and the discussion on the related methodological approach, as well as the case study related to immunization policy in the Gambia on which the methodological approach is based.

Definition

The World Health Organization (WHO, 2015) defines public health as all organized measures (whether public or private) to prevent disease, promote health, and prolong life among the population as a whole. Its activities aim to provide conditions in which people can be healthy and focus on entire populations, not on individual patients or diseases. Thus, public health is concerned with the total system and not only the eradication of a particular disease. Other definitions also circulate. For example, C.E.A Winslow (1920, cited by Merson et al 2006, p 13) frequently considered to be the founder of Public Health in the US characterizes public health as:

> the science and art of preventing disease, prolonging life and promoting physical health and efficiency through organized community efforts for the sanitation of the environment, the control of communicable infections, the education of the individual in personal hygiene, the organization of medical and nursing services for the early diagnosis and preventive treatment of disease, and the development of the machinery which will ensure to every individual a standard of living adequate for the maintenance of health; organizing these benefits in such a fashion as to enable every citizen to realize his birthright of health and longevity

These and other definitions of public health clearly relate to the many different ideas and images that the term public health invokes. These thoughts and descriptions include (Merson et al 2006): Is public health a discipline, a system, or a profession? Is it about providing clean water and sanitation, or functioning in an urban healthcare setting? Does it deal primarily with the health of the poor?

The dimensions of health that can encompass "a state of complete physical, mental and social well-being and not merely the absence of disease or infirmity", as defined by the WHO (1946), are often included in definitions of public health in response to these questions.

The term global public health acknowledges that, because of globalization, influences on public health can and do emerge from outside state boundaries and therefore responses to such public health issues currently demand attention to cross-border health risks, including change in the environment and accessing dangerous products (Merson et al 2006).

A Brief History

The history of international public health can be seen as a history of how political, social and economic systems create the chances for healthy or unhealthy lives; the manner in which populations experience wellness and illness; the manner in which individuals and groups try to prevent illness and promote their health; and the manner in which societies form the preconditions for the onset and spread of disease (Merson et al 2006). Among the many writers that have documented the history of public health Merson et al (2006) have presented a brief history to give a view of the difficulties we have to face, which is summarized in Box 1:

Box 1: A summarised History of International Public Health

400 BC	Hippocrates presented causal relationship between environment and disease
1st Century AD	Romans introduced public sanitation and organized water supply system
14th Century	Black Death led to quarantine and cordon sanitaire
Middle Ages	Colonial expansion spread infectious diseases around the world
1750-1850	Industrial Revolution resulted in extensive health and Social improvements in cities in Europe and the United States
1850- 1910	Great expansion of knowledge about the causes and trans mission of communicable diseases
1910-1945	Reduction in child mortality; establishments of schools of public health and international foundations and intergovern mental agencies interested in public health.
1945-1990	Creation of World Bank and other UN agencies; WHO eradicates smallpox; HIV/AIDs pandemic begins; Alma-Ata conference gives emphasis to primary health care; UNICEF leads efforts for universal childhood immunization; greater attention to chronic diseases
1990- 2005	Priority given to health sector reform, equity and development; impact of and response to globalization, cost-effectiveness, public-private partnerships in health, and use of information and communication technologies

Source: Merson et al (2006)

Facilitators

As Box 1 suggests, there are many facilitators of public health worldwide. They include accrediting bodies and organizations concerned about public health. For example, in a developed country like the US the National Network of Public Health Institutes (NNPHI) is a powerful force behind the execution of public health. This body supports public health accreditation and performance improvement through a variety of complimentary programmes, such as its Community of Practice for Public Health Improvement (COPPHI) programme whose activities are outlined in Box 2.

Box 2 : Community of Practice for Public Health Improvement (COPPHI) Programme

- COPPHI facilitates the exchange of best practices and builds capacity among the nation's health departments to become accredited and conduct quality improvement through the provision of grants, technical assistance, and shared learning opportunities.
- COPPHI reaches a broad range of local, state, and tribal health department representatives; researchers; public health institutes; universities; national public health organizations; funders; policymakers; and government agencies through the Open Forum for Quality Improvement in Public Health, the Kaizen Event Program, the Quality Improvement Award Program, the Gaining Ground Program, and the Public Health Quality Improvement Exchange.

Source: National Network of Public Health Institutes (2010)

In developing countries public health facilitators include public sector health systems that provide services to poor and marginalized populations. Such health systems face greater challenges than those in developed countries have to confront. In these poor countries institutions that are already fatigued by the effects of health sector reform and structural adjustment are frequently without much capacity and resources to deal with health burdens. Box 3 describes a strategic approach developed by the WHO, The Strategic Approach to Strengthening Reproductive Health Policies and Programmes, which facilitates public health in developing countries.

Box 3: The Strategic Approach to Strengthening Reproductive Health Policies and Programmes

The Strategic Approach to Strengthening Reproductive Health Policies and Programmes is a methodological innovation developed by the World Health Organization and its partners to help countries identify and prioritize their reproductive health service needs, test appropriate interventions, and scale up successful innovations to a sub national or national level. The participatory, interdisciplinary, and country-owned process can set in motion much-needed change.

The Strategic Approach was originally developed by the World Health Organization (WHO) and its partners to reorient the introduction of contraceptive methods from a technology-driven approach to one that is focused on quality of care and people's needs and rights. As countries began to apply the Strategic Approach during the 1990s, it was met with considerable enthusiasm. More and more governments requested assistance with applying the methodology. The Strategic Approach has now been implemented in 25 countries and has been adapted to be applicable for a range of reproductive health concerns

Source: Fajans et al (2006)

Characteristics

Selected unique features of public health has been defined as prevention (of deaths, illness, deaths, days lost from school or work, etc.), which is used as a major intervention strategy; grounding of public health in a multitude of sciences, including biostatistics, epidemiology, microbiology, economics, sociology, psychology and anthropology; social justice philosophy as a central pillar (its foundation is that the knowledge gained concerning how to ensure a health population should be shared equally among all societal groups); and links with government and public policy (governments design and implement public policy, and provide particular programmes and services) (Merson, et al 2006). However, as there are different public health systems, so also are varying public health characteristics. In the US, for example, public health systems consist of networks of state and local agencies that provide health care services to communities across the country (Mays et al 2009). Mays et al (2009) summarize what medical professionals know about the attributes of U.S. public health systems. They discuss organizational characteristics across four categories: 1) system boundaries and size; 2) organizational and inter organizational structures; 3) financing and economics; and 4) workforce characteristics. Box 4 presents these characteristics.

Box 4: Key attributes of U.S. public health systems

- State and local jurisdictions that define the boundaries of public health systems make it difficult to identify common tendencies.
- The use of local tax bases to support public health creates disparities in public health spending.
- What is known about efficiency and cost-effectiveness within public health systems relates to specific interventions rather than delivery systems as a whole.

Source: Mays et al (2009)

In Australia where, like in many developing countries, primary health care has been introduced, the characteristics of what is described as the new public health system (Box 5) seem comparatively more expansive and reflect the concept and principles of PHC.

Box 5: Characteristics of the New Public Health Approach
• Shift in focus to healthy public policy • Support for enhancement of life skills • Empowerment of individuals taking control of their health • Empowerment of communities to play an active role in setting health promotion, and developing and implementing health promotion strategies • Cooperation among health professionals and community members and organisations working together to promote health • A recognition of the social and environmental factors that determine health

BikiCrumba (2006)

Functions

The WHO states that there are three main public health functions:

The assessment and monitoring of the health of communities and populations at risk to identify health problems and priorities.

The formulation of public policies designed to solve identified local and national health problems and priorities.

Assuring that all populations have access to appropriate and cost-effective care, including health promotion and disease prevention services (WHO 2015)

These and other functions, such as the Essential Public Health Functions (EPHF) framework (WHO/PAHO (2000-2007) which has been in use for more than a decade, help countries define core public health functions and essential services to provide working definitions of public health and guiding framework for the responsibilities of public health systems. For example, in 1988, the Institute of Medicine (IOM) published a report, The Future of Public Health (Institute of Medicine 1988) that summarized a study undertaken to assess the status of public health in the United States. On the basis of the study findings, the IOM defined the mission of public health as fulfilling society's interest in assuring conditions in which people can be healthy. In regard to this mission, the IOM found that there are three core functions (responsibilities) of governmental public health agencies that are similar to the above three core functions identified by WHO: assessment, policy development, and assurance.

Similarly, in 1999 the Public Health in the Americas Initiative was launched as a partnership between the Latin American Center for Health Research

(CLAISS), the Centers for Disease Control and Prevention (CDC) and the Pan American Health Organization (PAHO)/World Health Organization (WHO). The goal of the Initiative was to establish the basis for achieving a regional commitment to strengthen public health in the Americas, including reaching a consensus on the concept of public health and its essential functions in the Americas, developing a methodology to measure EPHF performance, and offering support for the self-assessment of each country's public health status with respect to 11 defined Essential Public Health Functions (EPHF) (Box 6) and use the results obtained to carry out interventions to develop their capacity and improve public health practice.

Box 6: 11 Essential Public Health Functions

EPHF 1. Monitoring, evaluation, and analysis of health status
EPHF 2. Surveillance, research, and control of the risks and threats to public health
EPHF 3. Health promotion
EPHF 4. Social participation in health
EPHF 5. Development of policies and institutional capacity for public health planning and management
EPHF 6. Strengthening of public health regulation and enforcement capacity
EPHF 7. Evaluation and promotion of equitable access to necessary health services
EPHF 8. Human resources development and training in public health
EPHF 9. Quality assurance in personal and population-based health services
EPHF 10. Research in public health
EPHF 11. Reduction of the impact of emergencies and disasters on health

Source: WHO/PAHO (2000/2007)

Multidisciplinary teams of public health workers and professionals carry out the functions in Box 6 above. They include:

- Physicians specializing in public health/community medicine/infectious disease,
- Psychologists
- Epidemiologists,
- Biostatisticians,
- Medical assistants or Assistant Medical Officers,

- Public health nurses,
- Midwives,
- Medical microbiologists,
- Environmental health officers / public health inspectors,
- Pharmacists,
- Dental hygienists,
- Dietitians and nutritionists,
- Veterinarians,
- Public health engineers
- Public health lawyers,
- Sociologists and psychologists,
- Community development workers,
- Communications experts,
- Bioethicists,
- Sanitarians, occupational therapists and physical therapists
- Others

Concept Map

A concept map is a type of graphic organizer used to help organize and represent knowledge of a subject. Concept maps begin with a main idea (or concept) and then branch out to show how that main idea can be broken down into specific topics (Inspiration Software Inc., 2015). Health systems consist of all institutions, resources and organizations that take action primarily aimed at improving health (WHO, 2000). Health systems serve as the tools for carrying out the many public health functions we specified above. They crucially influence the degree to which countries are able to deal with their disease burden and improve the health of people generally as well as the health of specific groups (Merson et al, 2006)

In discussing the structuring of health systems conceptual maps, Merson et al (2006) dealt with the elements of health systems, typologies of health systems and evaluation of health systems.

Health System Elements

On the elements of health systems, Merson et al (2006) cite Roemer's (1991) five categories that can be used to carry out a detailed description of a country's health system. The categories are outlined in Box 7.

Box 7: WHO Health Systems Elements

- Service provision
- Resource generation(of inputs such as human resources and physical capital)
- Financing (revenue collection, pooling of resources, and purchasing health care)
- Stewardship (a broader concept than regulation, encompassing the necessary functions of government in safeguarding the health of its people)

Source: WHO (2000)

Although these classifications are helpful for describing health systems, they are less useful in understanding the performance of health systems. To be able to compare the performance of different health systems, it is necessary to group countries into a workable number of types (Merson et al, 2006).

Health System Typologies

According to Merson et al (2006) a more useful way of describing health systems was developed by the Organization for Economic Cooperation and Development (OECD) that includes not only the classification of economic aspects of health systems, but also the direction of reforms in health systems. The main classifications which are mostly relevant to developed countries, where the coverage of the health system consists of a few arrangements (OECD 1992, as cited by Merson et al 2006) are outlined in Box 8.

Box 8: OECD Classification of Health systems

- Whether the prime funding source consists of payments that are made voluntarily (as in private insurance or payment of user fees) or are compulsory (as in taxation or social insurance)
- Whether services are provided by direct ownership (termed the integrated pattern, where a ministry of health or social insurance agency provides services itself), by contractual arrangements (where a ministry of health or social insurance agency contracts with providers to deliver services,) or simply by private providers (paid by direct out-of-pocket payments)
- How services are paid for (prospectively, where financial risk is transferred to providers, or retrospectively, where the cost of care is reimbursed)

Source: OECD (1992), as cited by Merson et al (2006)

As already mentioned, health systems which, as the above description of health systems show, vary from country to country and influence the degree to which countries are able to deal with their disease burden and improve the health of people generally, as well as the health of specific groups (Merson et al, 2006). Therefore, public health systems do not equally share all of the key characteristics, defining criteria and antecedents and consequences this analysis covers.

For example, a huge disparity in access to health care and public health initiatives exist between developed nations and developing nations. In the developing world, public health infrastructures are still forming. In developing countries trained personnel and financial resources are often lacking. Even a basic level of medical care and disease prevention may not be available. The result is that a large majority of disease and mortality in the developing world results from and contributes to extreme poverty. For example, many African governments spend less than US$10 per person per year on health care, while, in the United States, the federal government spent approximately US$4,500 per capita in 2000.

However, public health plays an important role in disease prevention efforts in both the developing world and in developed countries, through local health systems and non-governmental organizations. The World Health Organization (WHO) is the international agency that coordinates and acts on global public health issues. In most countries there are government public health agencies, sometimes called ministries of health that deal with national or local health issues. One example is the frontline of public health initiatives in the US being state and local health departments. The public health service in this country is led by the Surgeon General, whiles the Centers for Disease Control and Prevention, based in Atlanta, is involved with several international health activities, in addition to its national duties. Another example is the Public health system in India that is managed by the Ministry of Health and Family Welfare of the government of India, but the health care facilities are state -owned.

Merson et al (2006) suggests that there is lack of a suitable typology for developing countries and presents a simple concept map (Figure 1) that indicates four main actors and four main functions needed in any health system.

Figure 1: A Map of the Health System

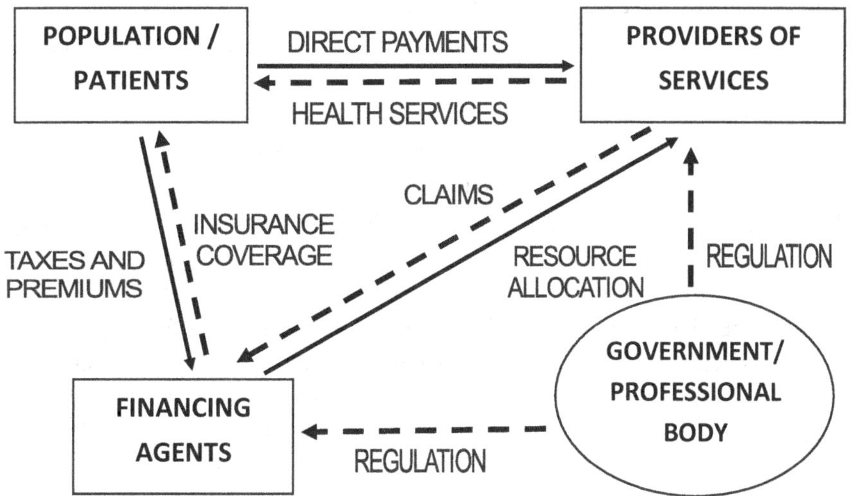

Source: Mills (2000b), as cited by Merson et al (2006)

The actors are:

- Governments or professional bodies that form and govern health systems
- Individuals and groups who pay for services they receive
- Financial agents who gather and allocate funds to service providers or buy services at the various levels of health care
- Providers of services at different levels of health care, working in curative or preventive care, in public or private health facilities, etc.

The functions are:

- Service provision
- Financing services through, for example, taxes
- Regulation
- Allocation of resources

The characteristics and activities of these actors are described in more detail in chapter 5 on the Resource map strategy

Health System Evaluation

Three main objectives of health systems have been proposed by the WHO (2000) as follows:

- To be responsive to peoples' expectations
- To be fair in financial contribution
- To ensure good health of individuals and groups

On the basis of these objectives the criteria of efficiency and equity are usually applied in assessing the performance of health systems (Merson et al 2006), as will be seen in following chapters. Efficiency consists of the following (Merson et al 2006):

Microeconomic efficiency- the extent for realizing more efficiency as a result of using existing resources. Microeconomic efficiency comprise *Allocative efficiency* (using resources for activities that have the greatest impact on health), and *Technical efficiency* (using only small amounts of resources on providing a specific activity or group of activities) *Macroeconomic efficiency*- total cost of the health system relative to total health status of populations. *Equity* – distributing the cost of health services and the gains from using the services among various groups in the population (Merson et al 2006). Equity is usually described in two ways (Donaldson et al1993): Horizontal equity (equal treatment of equals, for example, user fees should be the same for households with equal ability to pay) and, *Vertical equity* (people who are unequal in society should not be treated the same- consumers should be charged for the same services based on their ability to pay).

Several composite measures of health and disease have been used to measure the efficiency of health systems. Examples are healthy life years (HeaLY) and health-adjusted life expectancy (HALE). However, decisions grounded on the use of efficiency measures may not be suitable for measuring dimensions of equity (Merson et al, 2006)). Merson et al (2006) argue that "equity must be more than equality of access and must include a balance so that health system responses are in accord with equity as well as efficiency. They suggest that these summary indicators can be used as instruments for calculating healthy life per dollar to be realized by vulnerable and socioeconomic groups. Composite measures such as HeaLYs can be used not only for meeting efficiency criteria, but also to make sure that resources are distributed to those that need them most. Efficiency dimensions like cost-effectiveness are insufficient in guiding decisions on resource allocation; equity criteria should be combined with efficiency criteria to guide decision on distribution of resources (Merson et al, 2006).

Reidpath et al (2012, p8) argue that the idea of an equity-efficiency trade - off has incorrect thinking. They suggest that when one presupposes that the actual output of the system one is seeking is (a) known and agreed, and (b) not equity, one is assembling equity and efficiency in the way it is conventionally done in the literature. This, as they say, "leads to a paradox, because either we will fail to achieve the greatest quantum of the outputs that we really seek by diverting attention to unsought outputs in the domain of equity, or equity is a part of the outputs that we really seek, in which case there is no trade- off". Reidpath et al (2012) further argue that in order to discuss rationally the appropriate balance between the sought outputs of a health system, and the most efficient way of achieving those outputs, one should instead concentrate on the true trade off, between the different sought outputs (such as health gains and health equity)

Data for composite measures include:

- *Demographic data* for estimation of burden of disease
- *Mortality data* for analysis of burden of disease
- *Morbidity data* for estimation of, for example, the duration and severity of disability

These kinds of data should be processed in the form of particular disease-based estimates (variables), such as incidence rate. Again, the reader is referred to the wealth of information in the literature on such data for composite measures and the variables linked to them, such as (Merson et al 2006)).

The following chapters of this book illustrate the importance of using equity and efficiency criteria in assessing and understanding public health systems. As will be seen in these chapters, there is need to evaluate public health systems because of the need for evidence-based public health policy for, among other things:

- making decisions on the use of limited resources
- justifying action and demonstrating benefits of public health interventions
- informing politicians with limited health background who often make decisions

Related Concepts

The concepts most closely related to public health include community health, population health and Primary Health Care. In many countries community health and primary healthcare services now provide the contexts for delivery of public health programmes as means of achieving better health for the majority of people. A primary health care approach places emphasis on community-based services with increased attention on early intervention and prevention strategies such as health promotion. To be successful, community health programmes must depend on the dissemination of information by health professionals to the general public, using mass communication (one-to-one or one-to-many communication). Moreover, there is now a growing move towards health marketing (processes for creating, communicating, delivering, and exchanging offerings that have value for customers, clients, partners, and society at large) that combines traditional marketing principles and theories parallel with science-based strategies to prevention, health promotion and health protection (CDC 2011).

Community means a group of people who live in a defined geographical location and are governed by the same rules and regulations, norms, values, goals and organization. Its members are committed to interacting with each other broadly and honestly (Scott Peck et al, 1993). It can set standards for members and create the environment for great achievements (Manning et al, 1996)

The term community health means the health status of a defined group of people or community and the actions and conditions that protect and improve the health of the community (Green et al, 2002). For instance, the health status of people living in a particular village and the actions taken to protect and improve their health constitutes community health. However, due to contemporary quick modes of transportation, instant communication and the extending global economies, communities no longer have the resources to solely control or look after all the health needs of their residents without external help. Therefore, the term population health has been proposed (Green et al 2002). However, according to Kindig et al (2003, p 1), this term is relatively new and has not been properly defined. They propose this definition of population health: "The health outcomes of a group of individuals, including the distribution of such outcomes within the group". They argue that the field of population health should include patterns of health determinants and health outcomes, as well as policies and interventions that connect health determinants and health outcomes. Determinants of health include medical care systems (e.g. resource allocation and health interventions), the social environment (e.g. income, education and social support) and the physical surroundings (e.g. clean air and water, and urban design). Examples of health outcomes are length of life and health-related quality of life.

The term population health is similar to community health. The difference between population health and community health lies only in the scope of the people dealt with or the degree of organization (McKenzie et al 2011). The health statuses of populations who are not organized nor have no identity as a group or locality and the actions and conditions needed to protect and improve the health of these populations constitute population health (McKenzie et al, 2011). Examples of populations are women over fifty, adolescents, adults twenty-five to forty-four years of age, seniors living in public housing, prisoners, and blue-collar workers. It is clear from these examples that a population, as already mentioned, could be a segment of a community, a category of people in several communities of a region, or workers in various industries.

The Dahlgren and Whitehead (1991) Social Model of Health (Figure 2) is helpful for explaining the layers of influence on community/population health and discussing inequalities in health based on socioeconomic position. In discussing the layers of influence on health, Dahlgren and Whitehead (1991) outlined a social ecological theory to health. They try to map the relationship between individuals, their environment and disease.

Figure 2: Dahlgren and Whitehead Social Model of Health (1991)

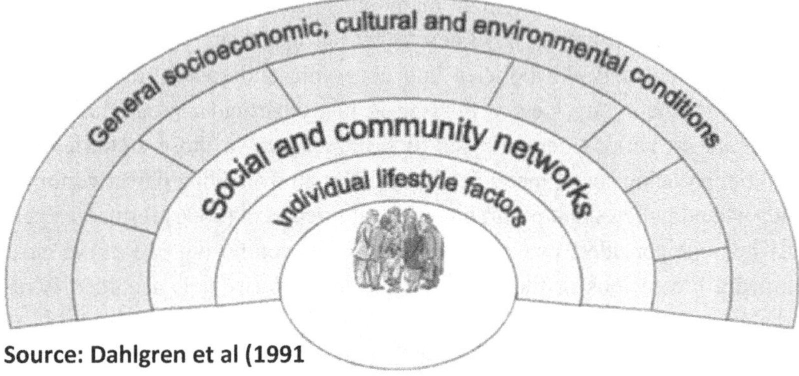

Source: Dahlgren et al (1991

The model shows the following influences on community/population health:
At the centre are individuals with a set of fixed genes. They are surrounded by influences on health that can be changed
First layer is personal behaviour and ways of living. These can promote or damage health, for example, choosing to drink alcohol or not. Here individuals are affected by friendship patterns and the norms of their community.
Second layer is social and community influences, which provide mutual support for members of the community in unfavourable conditions. But they can also fail to provide support or have a negative effect.
Third layer includes structural factors, namely, housing, working conditions, access to services and provision of essential facilities.

The model provides a useful framework for inquiring about the largeness of the contributions of each of the layers to health; the possibility of converting particular factors and the reciprocal actions needed to induce connected factors in other layers. Also, the model can be used for constructing several hypotheses on the inter-working between the different determinants of health, and the comparative influences of those determinants on various determinants (Public Health Action Support Group 2011).

In the introduction of their work entitled European Strategies for Tackling Social Inequities in health, Dahlgren et al (2006) point to this relationship between the individual, their environment and disease, and the unfairness of health inequities, which they say are caused by unhealthy public policies and lifestyles influenced by structural factors. They highlighted the importance given to efforts at reducing health inequities by an increasing number of countries and international bodies, such as the WHO, and the importance of improving health generally, especially in low-income countries, through attempts by countries and international agencies like the Commission on Social Determinants of Health (WHO 2008). Dahlgren et al (2006) also point out that despite such efforts; there still remain many gaps that need to be filled. As they indicate, very few countries have developed particular strategies for integrating equity-oriented health policies into economic and social policies. Also, they say that the equity view is missing in many particular programmes that concentrate on various determinants of health, “even in those countries that claim that reducing social inequities in health is an overriding objective for all health-related policies and programmes”. Dahlgren et al (2006) further suggest that when one considers that people see health as composing one of the most significant dimensions of their welfare, the low priority it is accorded is remarkable.

Community (and population) health in mainly the contexts of developing countries is usually studied and delivered based on the primary health care approach (e.g. Golladan (1980). Community Health Services play an important role in the primary health care system and aim to improve the health and well-being of people, especially people who are at risk of poorer health. Community health services give a strong stage for the delivery of a range of primary health care services, such as child health services. If delivered effectively, a PHC system can improve the health of a population and reduce inequalities in health care (Department of Health 2014). Thus, public health which focuses on population health and health inequalities is also closely related to PHC, a relationship that Boundris (2015, p 1) presents as follows:

[Primary health care is defined as] "an approach to health policy and service provision to individuals and populations that includes health services provided by both primary care and public health." Primary care is the first point of entry to a health care system, often a doctor or a nurse. Public health is an organized activity to promote, protect, improve, and restore the health of individuals, specified groups, or the population”. The reader is referred to the wealth of literature around community and population health and primary health care for further exploration of the terms and concepts. Examples are WHO (1978); WHO 2014; Bhatia et al (2010; Ruderman, M (2000); Green et al (1999; Boundris (2015))

Achievements

The most significant direct consequences and goal of public health include prevention and management of diseases, injuries and other health conditions through surveillance of cases and the promotion of healthy behaviours, communities and environments. The World Health Organization demonstrates the achievements of public health by drawing attention to the size of public health in terms of certain famous public health causes:

- Vaccination and control of infectious diseases
- Motor-vehicle safety
- Safer workplaces
- Safer and healthier foods
- Safe drinking water
- Healthier mothers and babies and access to family planning
- Decline in deaths from coronary heart disease and stroke
- Recognition of tobacco use as a health hazard (WHO 2015).

Box 9 presents in more detail these and other achievements of public health worldwide:

Box 9: Achievements of Public Health	
1.	**Vaccinations:** At the beginning of the 20th century, few effective treatments and preventive measures existed to prevent infectious diseases. However, vaccines have been developed and are used to prevent many of the infectious diseases that threatened our parents, grandparents, and great-grandparents during the 19th and early 20th century.
2.	**Safer workplaces:** At the beginning of the 20th century, workers in the United States faced remarkably high risks to their health and safety. Today, despite a much larger workforce than ever before, work-related deaths have declined sharply. Identifying and correcting occupational health hazards has greatly reduced the health and safety risks for such occupations as construction workers, miners, and farmers. For example, during 1933-1997, according to the National Safety Council, work-related injuries have declined 90%. And, although the workforce tripled during those years, deaths declined from 37/100,000 to 4/100,000 workers.
3.	**Safer and healthier foods:** Early in the 20th century, contaminated food, milk, and water were responsible for many food-borne diseases, including typhoid fever, tuberculosis, botulism, and scarlet fever. In the first half of the century, scientific discoveries and public health policies, such as food fortification programs, led to large reductions in diseases caused by nutritional deficiency. More recently, the focus of many public health nutrition programs shifted to the prevention and control of chronic disease, such as cardiovascular disease and obesity, through nutrition.

4.	**Motor-vehicle safety:** Although more people are driving automobiles, traveling more miles, and driving at faster speeds than in 1900, driving is much safer now because of safer vehicles, highways, and drivers. For example, since 1925, the annual death rate from motor-vehicle travel has decreased 90%. Systematic motor-vehicle safety efforts began during the 1960s. In 1966, passage of the Highway Safety Act and the National Traffic and Motor Vehicle Safety Act authorized the federal government to set and regulate standards for motor vehicles and highways, a mechanism necessary for effective prevention (2, 3). Other motor-vehicle safety successes include the following: • Approximately 85,000 American lives have been saved because of seat belts. • Using child safety seats has reduced the risk of infant death by 69% and by 47% for children aged 1 to 4 years. • Since 1987, community awareness and driving-while-intoxicated regulations have helped reduce alcohol related traffic fatalities by 32%.
5.	**Control of infectious diseases:** Public health action to control infectious diseases in the 20th century was founded on the late 19th century discovery of microorganisms as causes of many diseases. Further scientific findings documented the interactions among humans, the environment, and microbes. Improvements in sanitation and hygiene, food safety, the discovery of antibiotics, and the implementation of universal childhood vaccination programs resulted in the control of many fatal infectious diseases and the global eradication of one disease - smallpox. Scientific and technologic advances played a substantial role in the efforts. In addition, the discovery of antimicrobial therapy has contributed to the success of public health efforts to control various infections such as tuberculosis and sexually transmitted diseases. Today, those advances are the foundation for the disease surveillance and control systems that are used to combat all infectious diseases
6.	Decline in death from coronary heart disease and stroke: Since 1921, heart disease has been the leading cause of death, and since 1938, stroke has been the third leading cause of death. However, since 1950, age-adjusted death rates from cardiovascular disease (CVD) have declined 60%, representing one of the most important public health achievements in the 20th century. This decline was made possible through a better understanding of disease epidemiology and advances in prevention techniques, diagnoses, and treatment.

7.	**Family Planning:** During the 20th century, restrictive policies and laws affecting family planning were largely replaced by legislative and funding support for family planning services by physicians and specialized reproductive health-care providers. Modern contraception and reproductive health-care systems that became available later in the century further improved couples' ability to plan their families. Publicly supported family planning services prevent an estimated 1.3 million unintended pregnancies annually.
8.	**Recognition of tobacco use as a health hazard:** During the 20th century, smoking has gone from being an accepted norm to being recognized as the number one preventable cause of death and disability in the United States. Substantial public health efforts to reduce the prevalence of tobacco use began shortly after the risk was described in 1964. Although substantial progress has been made and millions of lives have been saved, increased prevention efforts are needed to reduce the impact of tobacco use on public health.
9.	**Healthier Mothers and Babies:** At the beginning of the 20th century, for every 1000 live births, 6-9 women in the United States died of pregnancy-related complications, and approximately 100 infants died before age 1 year. During 1915-1997, the infant mortality rate declined more than 90% to 7.2/1,000 live births, and during 1900-1997, the maternal mortality rate declined approximately 99% to <0.1 reported deaths/1,000 live births. These declines represent what many believe to be the most profound public health triumph of the 20th century. Many factors have contributed to this remarkable success story. Environmental interventions, improvements in nutrition, advances in clinical medicine, improvements in access to health care, improvements in surveillance and monitoring of disease, increases in education levels, and improvements in standards of living contributed to this remarkable decline.

10.	**Fluoridation of Drinking Water:** At the beginning of the 20th century, tooth decay was rampant, and because no effective preventive measures existed, tooth extraction was routine. Now, thanks to water fluoridation, combined with other dental health advances, adults in the United States are retaining most of their teeth throughout their lifetime. Fluoridation of community drinking water is a major factor responsible for the decline in dental caries (tooth decay) during the second half of the 20th century. The history of water fluoridation is a classic example of clinical observation leading to epidemiologic investigation and community-based public health intervention. Water fluoridation remains the most equitable and cost-effective method of delivering fluoride to all members of most communities, regardless of age, educational attainment, or income level.

Source: CDC (1999)

Operational Definition

Scott et al (2009) define the term operational definition as the transformation of a theoretical concept, an abstract, into something tangible, observable, concrete, and measurable in an empirical research project. Here we adapt the World Health Organization's (WHO 2015) definition of public health as including the following: (1) all organized measures (whether public or private) to prevent disease, promote health, and prolong life among the population as a whole and (2), activities that aim to provide conditions in which people can be healthy and focus on entire populations, not on individual patients or diseases. Thus, public health is concerned with the total system and not only the eradication of a particular disease.

Challenges of Public Health

Despite the many achievements of public health outlined above, there are many challenges that have been well-described in the literature. While many writers have focused on country specific challenges, others (e.g. Myerson et al 2006) have looked at universal public health challenges particularly at the start of the 21st Century. These challenges include (Merson et al 2006):

- Preventable causes of death such as malaria and diarrhea
- Limited access to contraceptive for limitation of childbearing
- Death from complications of pregnancy
- Death from mostly preventable or curable infectious diseases
- Lack of access to clean water
- Increased risk for non-communicable diseases, such hypertension and

diabetes, due to factors such as obesity.

- Poverty which is an important underlying cause of disease, etc.
- Human migration, displacement, bioterrorism, and disaster preparedness

There are many national and international declarations aimed at tackling such public health challenges. Perhaps the most important of these are the Millennium Development Goals. Box 10 lists the MDGs that were adopted by the UN General Assembly in September 2000 as a set of key objectives and guiding principles for international collaboration.

Box 10: Millennium Development Goals	
	Goal 1: Eradicate Extreme Hunger and Poverty
	Goal 2: Achieve Universal Primary Education
	Goal 3: Promote Gender Equality and Empower Women
	Goal 4: Reduce Child Mortality
	Goal 5: Improve Maternal Health
	Goal 6: Combat HIV/AIDS, Malaria and other diseases
	Goal 7: Ensure Environmental Sustainability
	Goal 8: Develop a Global Partnership for Development

Source: UNDP (2006)

As can be seen, goals 4, 5 and 6 particularly refer to health. The resources that are required to realize these and the other goals have been outlined by the

WHO Commission on Macroeconomics and Health (WHO 2001), and have been later refined by Sachs et al (2005). Meeting the MDGs require international and inter-sectoral cooperation between UN agencies and other international bodies and philanthropists in health, such as Bill Gates. As Merson et al (2006) suggest, guaranteeing the ideal establishment and proper functioning of this world-wide health system is another huge challenge for public health in the next decade and beyond. Box 11 outlines several challenges to realizing the MDGs (Abaza 2003)

Box 11: Challenges to Realizing the Millennium Development Goals

... *the Millennium Development Goals* strongly influence the focus and direction of much of the development assistance activities of the multilateral organizations and bilateral agencies. There are three main challenges to realizing the *Millennium Development Goals.* First, to the extent possible, actions to achieve one of the goals should not compromise the ability to achieve any of the other goals. This requires the ability not only to assess the outcome of actions to achieve a certain goal, but also the positive and negative impacts of the intended action on the ability to achieve any of the other goals. Basically, it is an issue of ensuring the most cost-effective allocation of resources during the economic development of a country.

The second challenge relates to a potentially important weakness in the design and delivery of poverty alleviation programmes. The focus on poverty alleviation has engendered a strong emphasis on the delivery of economic benefits to the poorest people on the basis that a higher standard of living will also improve health and educational opportunities (*both Millennium Development Goals*). However, the assumption that any strategy, programme or set of actions aimed at poverty alleviation is also environmentally sustainable is debatable. Thus, it is imperative that efforts are made to incorporate environmental considerations into poverty alleviation programmes.

Finally, the *Millennium Development Goal* that each country should integrate the principles of sustainable development into country policies and programmes (for example, through implementation of a National Strategy for Sustainable Development) present a major opportunity as well as a challenge. Achieving this goal will reinforce the need to use an integrated, cross-sectoral and comprehensive approach to ensure sustainability aspects are incorporated into policy design and decision-making.

There has been much debate on why the MDGs as they relate to maternal and infant mortality rates, for instance, have not been met in the fifteen years they were to be realized. For example, during this period there have been 50% infant mortality rates in some developing countries. Although there are measurement problems such as inadequate and unreliable data, such deaths are attributable to several resource, managerial, policy and environmental factors, such as lack of equipment, material and drugs; limited and inadequately trained health staff, low staff motivation linked to poor working conditions, etc; high disease burden, weak economies and poor health financing; and weak health infrastructure.

The MDGs were supposed to be achieved by 2015, so a further process was needed to agree and develop development goals from 2015-2030, the Sustainability Development Goals. On 25 September 2015, countries were given the opportunity to adopt this set of global goals to end poverty, protect the planet, and ensure prosperity for all as part of a new sustainable development agenda (UN 2015). Each goal (Box 12) has specific targets to be achieved over the next 15 years.

Box 12: Sustainability Development Goals

- End poverty in all its forms everywhere[12]
- End hunger, achieve food security and improved nutrition and promote sustainable agriculture
- Ensure healthy lives and promote well-being for all at all ages
- Ensure inclusive and equitable quality education and promote lifelong learning opportunities for all
- Achieve gender equality and empower all women and girls
- Ensure availability and sustainable management of water and sanitation for all
- Ensure access to affordable, reliable, sustainable and modern energy for all
- Promote sustained, inclusive and sustainable economic growth, full and productive employment and decent work for all
- Build resilient infrastructure, promote inclusive and sustainable industrialization and foster innovation
- Reduce inequality within and among countries
- Make cities and human settlements inclusive, safe, resilient and sustainable
- Ensure sustainable consumption and production patterns
- Take urgent action to combat climate change and its impacts
- Conserve and sustainably use the oceans, seas and marine resources for

sustainable development
- Protect, restore and promote sustainable use of terrestrial ecosystems, sustainably manage forests, combat desertification, and halt and reverse land degradation and halt biodiversity loss
- Promote peaceful and inclusive societies for sustainable development, provide access to justice for all and build effective, accountable and inclusive institutions at all levels
- Strengthen the means of implementation and revitalize the global partnership for sustainable development

Source: United Nations (2015)

The importance of the MDGs (and the new SDGs) in sustainability assessment of public health policy change is demonstrated by its use as a reference for impact assessment (e.g., International Working Group 2006; Abaza 2003) which, as indicated, includes sustainability impact assessment. For example, to assess the impact and sustainability of small-scale renewable energy projects in developing countries the International Working Group for Monitoring and Evaluation in Energy for Development (M&EED) suggests that the MDGs should be used as reference in assessment as they represent the international priorities for sustainable development. The researchers as a result assessed the findings of the evaluation based on their contribution to realizing the MDGs (International Working Group 2006). As the following chapters show, the MDGs or SDGs are now recurring themes in the public health policy literature.

Implications for Research and Practice

The extent to which public health practitioners identify and help implement strategies for improving the health of an entire population group can affect the quality of public health services. As we have seen in the foregoing discussion, public health gives various values and tools to approach health care, such as emphasizing prevention, using and expanding the science base, seeking social equity, and building partnerships. While the benefits of public health worldwide are unquestionable, there appears to be relatively little results in the area of public health research, at least in developing regions of the world like Africa. For example, a WHO/African Region (WHO/AFRO) study (Nachega et al, 2012) has shown that little has been published about epidemiology and public health capacity, including research, in WHO/AFRO to help guide future planning by various stakeholders. The authors conclude that although since 1991, there has been increasing epidemiological research productivity in WHO/ AFRO that is linked to the number of epidemiology programmes and burden of HIV/AIDS cases, more capacity building and training initiatives in epidemiology are needed to promote research and deal with the public health challenges facing the continent. Figure 3 shows the relationship between research evidence and decisions for public health practice.

Figure 3: The Relationship between research evidence and decisions for public health practice

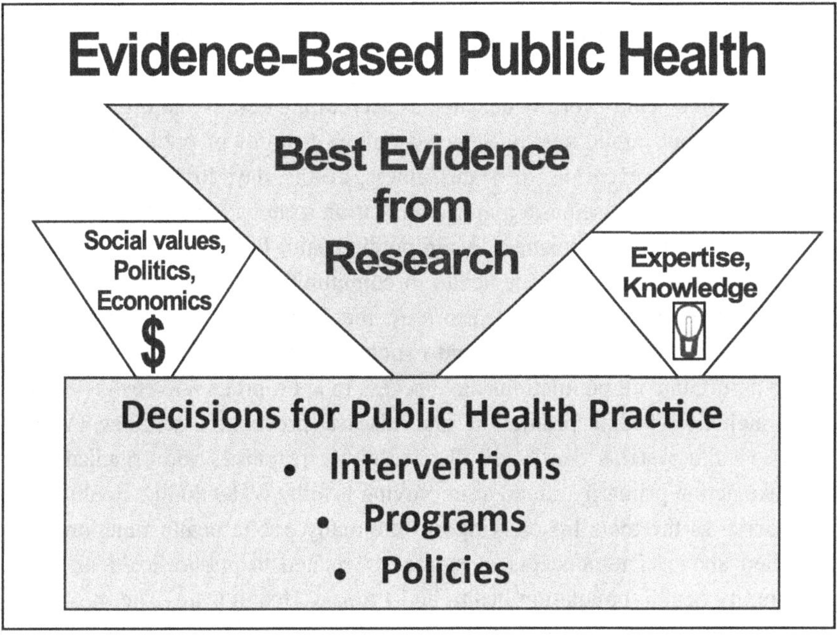

Source: Medical Research Library of Brooklyn (2004)

As Figure 3 demonstrates, the public health value of using and expanding the science base serves to ensure that decision making is data driven, and that research and demonstrations that enhance scientific knowledge are encouraged and supported. Public health professionals have always been doing things in a certain ways - common practice without research to back them up. Public health professionals need to prove or provide evidence to back up decisions about the use of resources, etc. Furthermore, politics overlay decision-making on everything that is not evidence-based in the public health world. Everything public health professions do is affected by political priorities and funding decisions. Therefore, the importance of providing best evidence from research to influence decisions for public health practice cannot be overemphasized.

Francis Sarr

Summary

Public health can be defined as all organized measures (whether public or private) to prevent disease, promote health, and prolong life among the population as a whole. Its activities aim to provide conditions in which people can be healthy and focus on entire populations, not on individual patients or diseases. The history of international public health can be seen as a history of how political, social and economic systems create the chances for healthy or unhealthy lives; the manner in which populations experience wellness and illness; the manner in which individuals and groups try to prevent illness and promote their health; and the manner in which societies form the preconditions for the onset and spread of disease (Merson et al 2006). There are many facilitators of public health worldwide, such as accrediting bodies and organizations concerned about public health. Selected unique features of public health has been defined as prevention (of deaths illness, deaths, days lost from school or work, etc.), which is used as a major intervention strategy; grounding of public health in a multitude of sciences. Main public health functions include the assessment and monitoring of the health of communities and populations at risk to identify health problems and priorities; the formulation of public policies designed to solve identified local and national health problems and priorities; and to assure that all populations have access to appropriate and cost-effective care, including health promotion and disease prevention services (WHO 2015). Health systems consist of all institutions, resources and organizations that take action primarily aimed at improving health (WHO 2000). Health systems serve as the tools for carrying out the many public health functions we specified above. The concepts most closely related to public health include community health, population health and Primary Health Care. The most significant direct consequences and goal of public health include prevention and management of diseases, injuries and other health conditions through surveillance of cases and the promotion of healthy behaviours, communities and environments. Despite the many achievements of public health, there are many challenges that need to be tackled now and in the future, including guaranteeing the ideal establishment and proper functioning of the international and inter-sectoral cooperation between UN agencies and other international bodies and philanthropists in health. Public health gives various values and tools to approach health care, such as emphasizing prevention, using and expanding the science base, seeking social equity, and building partnerships. However, there appears to be relatively little results in the area of public health research, at least in developing regions of the world like Africa. More capacity building and training initiatives in epidemiology are needed to promote research and deal with the public health challenges facing the African continent and other parts of the world. The following chapter deals with the concept of sustainability in public health which is widely considered a major challenge confronting public health in especially developing countries, but a main theoretical contributor to the SIA framework and the case study.

2

Sustainability

It has been suggested that public health programmes can only deliver benefits if they are able to sustain activities over time (Schell et al, 2013). As will be seen in this chapter, this is one of many proposals on how public health programmes can or should be sustained. Furthermore, the sustainability term itself evokes various ideas and images. As Schell et al further suggest the wide literature on programme sustainability in public health is in pieces and there is a lack of consensus on core constructs. The purpose of this chapter is to present an analysis of the concept of sustainability to improve general clarity and comprehension of the concept as it applies to public health, the Sustainability Impact Assessment framework and the case study that illustrates the SIA's role in public health policy change. It begins with a definition of the term sustainability.

Definition

There are different views about what *sustainability* means and what can be done to foster it. However, *sustainability* is generally seen as an economic, social and ecological concept. For example, a definition that emphasizes public policy approaches defines sustainability as the "satisfaction of basic economic, social, and security needs now and in the future without undermining the natural resource base and environmental quality on which life depends" (WCED 1987, p.3). Other definitions stress the maintenance of programmes at a certain level or rate, the continuation of programmes, and routinization and standardization processes (Christopher et al, 2013). Christopher et al (2013, p 3) suggest that such definitions indicate an overgeneralization and redefinition of sustainability "simply as organizational survival, divesting it from its focus on environmental protection and minimizing the classic ecological dilemma..."

However, in public health programmes like immunization, for instance, because of the nature of immunization and the international interest in the success of immunization programmes, the focus of sustainability has moved from the narrow meaning provided by the United Nations World Commission on Environment and Development (WCED 1987) towards a broader concept - the ability of a country to mobilize and allocate sufficient domestic and external resources on a reliable basis to achieve target levels of immunization performance.

A definition that captures the main essential elements of these definitions of the term sustainability in the context of the EPI is provided in The Common Assessment Tool for Immunization Services (WHO 2002): *the ability of an organization to provide quality service to its clients, increase or maintain demand for services, expand services to reach people who are not currently reached and generate financial resources.*

The case study example (Chapters 7-10) and the Sustainability Impact Assessment framework on which the book is based are contingent on the three pillars of sustainable development: economic, environmental and social sustainability. However, as the above definitions show, visions of sustainable development are evolving, particularly when governments strive to establish sustainable development strategies and wish to integrate fully sustainability in all policy development. Some countries adopt a more integrated approach that goes beyond the idea of the three pillars and encompasses systemic and systematic sustainable development goals for policy development (in line with, for instance, Agenda 21 adopted at the 1992 United Nations Conference on Environment and Development— the Earth Summit (OECD 2010)

Sustainability Issues

Three current social, financing and environmental sustainability debates/ issues and how they relate to the case study are outlined in the following sections, as examples of issues that specifically relate to or precede sustainability in public health. These issues are ethics, the global marketplace and healthcare financing, including the issues of structural adjustments and governance as they concern sustainability in health care in general and the EPI in particular.

Social sustainability: Ethics

This includes:

- Ethical concerns for future generations, as well as legal rights for future generations.
- Ethical concerns for non-human organisms and natural ecosystems (Columbia University, 2005).
- The belief that scientific knowledge can influence cultural ethics, and that there is a degree of mutuality between religious and scientific systems.
- The belief that ethical systems can provide the foundation of an environmental ethic (Columbia University, 2005).
- The view that social equity is also a principle of sustainability, since the wellbeing of individuals and the stability of society are crucial to creating a stable world (Columbia University, 2005). Social equity includes eliminating poverty so that everyone has his/her basic needs met. Such basic needs include clean water, adequate food, sanitation, shelter, the opportunity to earn a living, and access to health care (Columbia University, 2005).

In the case study, such ethical issues are addressed in relation to several questions. The study seeks to find out, among other things, whether the EPI is able to sustain demand and reduce barriers to accessing immunization through strategies like public information, social mobilization and identification of critical barriers to immunization.

Environmental sustainability: Global Marketplace

This includes:

- Ecological sustainability. One category aims primarily at sustaining human welfare, whereas the other aims at preserving ecosystems integrity.
- Concerns about various practices and philosophies in the world today as being inimical to sustainability, for example, the philosophy of infinite economic growth and infinite growth in consumption are completely unsustainable and will cause great harm to human civilization in the future.
- A growing awareness that there must be limits to certain kinds of human activity if life on the planet is to survive indefinitely (Goodland et al1996, Albright 1997).
- Concerns about the dramatic pace of globalization; that there has been a remarkable increase in the flow of capital from the developed to the developing countries due to increased private investment (Goodland et al, 1996); that the environmental impacts of these flows are high because the North is investing little in sustainability in the developing nations but is

continuing the old types of "resource intensive growth" and mining natural capital; that organizations like the Global Alliance for Vaccines and Immunization (GAVI) are using their power to force individual countries to prioritize in the way that suits them.

Assessment of the expansion of the sustainability of the EPI by this case study necessitated a look at how the activities of external donors are affecting the financial sustainability of the EPI, particularly in terms of the impact of the introduction of new vaccines. Particularly, the study tried to find out whether the country is able to sustain the introduction of new vaccines in a climate of decreasing donor support, and the consequences of unsustainable introduction of vaccines for the immunization system.

Health care financing

Financial sustainability of the general health sector

This includes:

- The realization by developing countries that the priorities of donors are subject to a variety of forces: geopolitical changes have been shown to elevate the importance of providing new or additional aid to one set of countries, while diminishing the emphasis of giving aid to others.
- Changing donor priorities as one school of thought about the process of development gives ground to another.
- New understandings of the causes of diseases and the problems inherent in health systems—and new conceptual frameworks and methodologies for identifying priorities—have had dramatic implications for the types of interventions that donors seek to support. Sustainability has become synonymous with self-sufficiency
- Several strategies being employed to develop long-term financial support for health systems, diversifying sources of financing away from external aid, such as establishment of efficiency - and equity-based criteria for public sector spending; the introduction of user fees, the introduction of efficiency measures to reduce the costs of service delivery; the promotion of risk-pooling and private financing through community-based and other forms of health insurance; and greater private sector participation in the financing and delivery of clinical services, and a corresponding reduction in the burden on the public sector (Levine et al 2001).

The efforts of such basic health services have generally been successful, with some health centres running surpluses and others requiring ongoing external support, though their broader impact on quality of care and community responsiveness has been generally positive (Levine et al., 2001).

- The realization that although it is relatively easy to see the dangers for immunization programmes of high levels of dependence on external aid and thus the imperative to increase the commitment of developing country governments, the traditional "self-sufficiency" arguments work less well for immunization than for many other health services. This is because immunization financing does not lend itself to some of the strategies typically employed to foster sustainability; short-term, unpredictable fluctuations in financing for immunization programmes have a disproportionate impact; funding requirements to achieve optimum health benefits may increase quickly, while the political culture in developing countries may be slow to change; some long-term international support may be justified on the basis of global externalities; some level of long-term international support may be justified on the basis of equity objectives. Therefore, self-sufficiency is not considered the objective that underpins financial sustainability plans (Levine et al., 2001).

Structural adjustments, governance and sustainability in health care

These include:

- The events that led to the economic crisis of the 1980's which were generally the flow of credit to the Third World, repeated increases in oil prizes and thereafter, interest rates that produced huge debts in those countries, recession in the industrialized nations and low commodity prices globally. These factors affected national incomes and resulted in huge government budget deficits.
- Adjustment and stabilization packages during the 1980s are which were initiated in most developing countries. Such packages or polices that are commonly known as Structural Adjustment Policies (SAPS) aimed at strengthening the balance of payments, opening up to the world market, and reducing the state's role in economic planning and the provision of social services.
- Differing consequences of the seriousness of the economic conditions in developing countries and the content, scope and timing of these adjustment measures, as did the consistency and degree of their implementation (Streefland et al., 1995).
- The recognition that while the impact of SAPS on health and health status has been positive, in poor countries economic decline and SAPS have contributed to impoverishment at the household level on the one hand, and to poor functioning of basic health services in the periphery and the

collapse of community-based health care on the other (Streefland et al 1995), and serious negative effects on welfare (Costello et al., 1994).

- The economic crisis leading donor governments to insert economic values—such as cost-recovery and financial sustainability—into their health assistance schemes. Selective vertical programmes enabled international aid agencies to measure results and protect their financial investments from complicated, long-term, multisectoral, and interdepartmental implementation procedures.
- NGOs and religious groups finding that holistic community-based health programmes are generally undermined by narrowly selective interventions and that the sustainability of people-owned initiatives can be put in jeopardy.
- Bilateral donors being uneasy about satisfying their taxpaying constituencies that overseas development assistance was being well spent. They became impatient at the slow pace of the processes of community participation necessary for strategies like primary health care to succeed (Macfarlane et al., 2000).
- The more authoritarian governments in developing countries looked upon community empowerment, management, and demand processes as forces likely to undermine their control, not only over health but, ultimately, the entire political system; hence, they had little or no interest in fostering such democratic outcomes. Nor, in another version of reordered power relations, were national governments willing to foster local government autonomy.
- Government bureaucracies—whether at national or local levels—being simply unaccustomed or unwilling to work as peers with people at the community level and therefore finding it difficult to develop the needed institutional mechanisms (Macfarlane et al., 2000).
- The expectation that health systems, like other public entities, are expected to become efficient in the management of revenue and expenditure, the administration of services and the enablement of government, the private sector and communities to contribute to better health care. Issues of efficient governance (including accountability) have been addressed by a set of joint practices of collaboration between public and private bodies at various levels, including public-private partnerships, contractual procedures and co-funding mechanisms (United Nations, 2001). Experiences in the developing world in health care illustrate the benefits of such innovations.
- Concerns about how to foster long-term sustainability by broadening con-

sultation mechanisms and allowing maximum participation at the local level, which is likely to promote efficiency and productivity, improve service delivery and increase production and resource mobilization and accountability and transparency through practical means such as transparent tendering procedures and independent auditing

- Advocates of health-sector reform recognizing the need not only for "community participation" but also for "consumer responsiveness" (Macfarlane et al., 2000), including the poor.

The case study (Chapters 7-10) attempts to use indicators of financial sustainability of immunization programmes (Levine et al 2001) under the dimensions of a system that has stable financing at a level that permits the achievement of coverage targets. Through the use of a set of indicators the study seeks to find out which actions to improve efficiency in the supply chain and reliable and sufficient funding for the EPI do key stakeholders support and the extent to which they think actions have been taken or implemented by government. Also, with the help of a resource map framework the study describes the flow and uses of funds in the immunization system, as well as compiling data that focus on questions of power, relationships, processes and accountability in the EPI.

Characteristics of Sustainability

Comprehensive reviews of the literature have attempted to identify the defining attributes of sustainability. For example, Schell et al (2013) identify 85 relevant studies focusing on programme sustainability in public health, including prevention-oriented programmes aimed at the community level. The concept-mapping process provided critical descriptors that elicited a mental image of the idea of sustainability in public health. According to the review, for sustainability to be present there must be: (1) Political Support; (2) Funding Stability; (3) Partnerships; (4) Organizational Capacity; (5) Programme Evaluation; 6) Programme Adaptation; (7) Communications; (8) Public Health Impacts, and (9) Strategic Planning.

However, as we have seen, the domains and items that constitute sustainability and the emphasis placed on them can be less or more than the ones specified above depending on the different conceptualizations of sustainability. For example Christopher et al (2013) would rather give more importance to programme effectiveness and responsiveness to public health needs rather than on their financial viability. Box 13 presents a more detailed conceptualization of sustainability outcomes by Scheirer et al (2011) in terms of six types of dependent variables that emphasize this important sustainability element.

Box 13: Conceptualization of sustainability outcomes in terms of 6 types of potential dependent variables

1. Whether benefits or outcomes for consumers, clients, or patients are continued (when the intervention provides services to individuals).

This individual-level dependent variable requires that an information system continues to capture at least the volume of services provided to consumers. Even better would be continued documentation of changed behavioral or clinical outcomes among clients, if a data system is available to provide evidence of the intended continued effects among clients. Continued achievement of client benefit after external funding stops can be realized if stakeholders are aware of the benefits achieved and they address the business-as-usual difficulties of their achievement (Steadman et al 2002; Blasinsky et al 2006).

2. Continuing the program activities or components of the original intervention.

This issue has been the focus of much previous research and is a legitimate dependent variable for this line of research. Rather than being phrased as a dichotomy—"Did the program continue or not?"—the research would be more explicit by enumerating the components of the intervention and inquiring about the extent to which each component is continued (Scheirer 2008). This type of operationalization would thus build on work in implementation science (Damschroder et al 2009; Century et al 2010) by first distinguishing manifest program components (e.g., trained coaches, written intervention protocols, interagency collaborative review) from the theoretical components or constructs that underlie the intervention (e.g., stages of change, self-efficacy, or behavioral reinforcement theories).

Ideally, the program developers and researchers would have tested and differentiated the manifest program components as operationalization of either core manifest components (those program structures and processes that causally lead to observed desired outcomes) or customizable manifest components that implementers can be encouraged to modify without logical or actual harm to the effectiveness of the intervention. Adaptations of the customizable components may contribute to the host organization's or community's identification with the program; for instance, through modifications to the language for branding the intervention and communicating with its intended beneficiaries, use of images that closely mirror a particular new target population's demographics, or additional steps or resources that a particular adopting organization has at its disposal. This specification and measurement of the activities or components defining the program links sustainability with the previous stages in an overall life cycle of intervention development, adoption, implementation (with potential iterative adaptations), and sustainability (Scheirer 1999; Rovniak et al 2005; Dearing 2009).

3. Maintaining community-level partnerships or coalitions developed during the funded programme.

Programs that came about as a result of formal community coalitions may see the continuance of the coalition after the initial program funding ends, even if the coalition does not continue all the specific program-level activities they implemented during the funded period. The community's readiness and capacity for interagency communication, cooperation, and collaboration may be a valuable sustained outcome that could lead to a new set of activities or benefits for consumers (Dearing et al 2010). Sometimes coalitions spin off programs as social or policy entrepreneurs by encouraging others to adopt a program or vesting a coalition program with its own scaled-up staff and organization. Maintaining the broader community capacity for change could lead to changes in the social environment that ultimately create population-wide benefits. Participants in our discussions of these issues emphasized that maintaining community-level partnerships is important to longer-term work on the focus issue, even if the activities of a specific program are not continued.

4. Maintaining new organizational practices, procedures, and policies that were started during program implementation.

Sustainability researchers have long recognized that the extent to which a host organization or partner organization changes its practices, procedures, and policies within its operations and structure can be an important reflection of degree of program institutionalization (Goodman et al 1993). Yet sustained change in organizational policies or procedures could be an important outcome in itself, whether or not other program activities remain. For example, starting up and sustaining a no-smoking policy in a workplace would be an important outcome, even if other components from a broader smoking-cessation program were not sustained in that location.

5. Sustaining attention to the issue or problem.

A valued outcome of program implementation, especially in high-profile efforts, is general heightened issue salience. Social problems that continue to be recognized as public issues through sustained organizational resources and sustained media coverage can lead to public perceptions of increased issue severity, as well as policymakers paying greater policy attention to the issue and allocating more resources to it (Dearing et 2010). Researchers studying sustainability can often identify valid longitudinal archival indicators of issue salience in media, public, and policy agendas that reflect the activity and successes of issue proponents, media advocates, and policy entrepreneurs.

6. Programme diffusion and replication in other sites.

Another potential longer-term outcome from worthy innovative programmes is that the underlying concepts or interventions themselves may spread to other locations (Weiss 1997; Rogers 2003). The innovation, including the ideas or principles upon which it is based, may diffuse into use at other locations even if it is not maintained in the initial location. The extent of dissemination activities by staff or proponents of the initial programme is an indirect proxy indicator for this type of potential sustainability outcome, although such dissemination itself does not measure the actual extent of adoption or implementation of a programme by other agencies or communities. Dissemination activities are conceptually distinct from and logically antecedent to subsequent diffusion into actual use (Dearing et 2010). Further detailed research is needed to assess whether, and under what conditions, dissemination activity by programme staff or a sponsoring change agency does in fact lead decision-makers in other organizations or communities to notice, try, adopt, implement, and sustain the same or adapted versions of public health programmes.

A Generic Conceptual Framework for Sustainability

Scheirer et al (2011) have formulated a generic conceptual framework for sustainability which is very much reflective of the conceptual framework in the case study described in chapters 7-10. According to Scheirer et al, although this framework does not include all the factors that may be important in a particular context, it indicates that financial sources are hypothesized as intervening variables between the different set of factors influencing sustainability and potential longer-term sustainability outcomes. Scheirer et al say that in this conceptualization, continued financial support is not synonymous with sustainability, but the availability of resources is hypothesized as a key influence on sustainability outcomes.

Scheirer et al (2011) explain that all of these processes take place in an encompassing broader context: the social, policy, and financial environments (underlying potential sources for funding in support of interventions of a specific type, such as whether foundations emphasize smoking cessation or obesity prevention, or whether government agencies provide funding for specific types of interventions). As Schell et al (2013) suggest, sometimes the contextual factors may prove to be the principal influences on sustaining public health programmes, particularly when internal organizational and community supports that might normally underpin sustainability find it difficult to deal with major changes in these environmental forces.

Thus, this generic conceptual framework is in many ways consistent with the case study conceptual framework which focuses on similar contextual factors that influence the sustainability of the EPI. This framework demonstrates that the issue of sustainability of the EPI cannot be divorced from the political and economic climate surrounding a health programme, both in the local context, and in the wider national and international context. Some of the most common influences or threats to the sustainability of the EPI are shown in Figure 6, chapter 8. As Figure 6 shows, threats to the sustainability of the EPI in relation to the country and its government, for example, are government bureaucratic procedures, poor economic conditions in the country, currency devaluation and unfavourable political climate.

Facilitators

The above discussion demonstrates that many organizational, environmental, social and other factors facilitate sustainability in public health. For example (Edvardsson et al 2011), facilitators as experienced by professionals involved in a multi-sectoral child health programme included being actively involved in intervention development and small-scale testing, personal values corresponding to programme intentions, regular meetings, working close with collaborators, using manuals and a clear programme branding. In other words, facilitating factors include involving front-line professionals in intervention development and using small scale testing, as well as paying attention to the role of managerial support and an overall supportive system. The importance for both practitioners and researchers to pay attention to parallel processes at different levels in multidisciplinary improvement efforts that are aimed at ensuring sustainability is emphasized.

Sustaining important public or grant-funded services after initial funding is terminated or reduced significantly is a major public health challenge. The case study described in Chapters 7-10 focuses on such an issue in the EPI by investigating the sustainability question of whether the country which is experiencing inconsistent donor funding and the effects of a weak economy can afford new vaccines or whether it should mobilize the limited funds to reach more children. LaPelle et al (2006) describe a similar example to demonstrate different levels of achieving sustainability: programmes with high sustainability, programmes with moderate sustainability, and programmes with no sustainability. The researchers in this example investigated whether tobacco treatment services previously funded within a statewide tobacco control initiative could be sustained after state funding was terminated abruptly. They found that two key strategies—redefining the scope of services being offered and creative use of resources—were factors that determined whether some community agencies were able to sustain services at a much higher level than others after funding was discontinued. They suggest that understanding these strategies and developing them at a time when programme funding is not being threatened is likely to increase programme sustainability.

In addition to such existing sustainability efforts are more recent references like the USA Environmental Protection Agency http://www.epa.gov (and EPA's Health Impact Assessments (HIA)) that are important facilitators of sustainability in public health.

Related Concepts

The concepts most connected to sustainability as it relates to public health include sustainable development, sustainable growth, social sustainability and its related concepts of human and social capital, and self-sufficiency. The original term of sustainability is sustainable development (UNCED 1992). Some experts now object to the term sustainable development as an umbrella term since it implies continued development that will cause great harm to humans in the future. In contrast, sustainability integrates environmental, economic and social concerns. Sustainability, then, is nowadays applied as a criterion to evaluate all aspects of human activity.

In economics, sustainable growth consists of increases in real incomes (i.e. "Inflation" -adjusted) or output that could be sustained for long periods of time (Department for the Environment, Food and Rural Affairs 2009). So, sustainable growth means, among other things, making profit.

Social sustainability is concerned with the maintenance of social and human capital and keeping social and human capital intact. Human capital consists of knowledge, disposition, skills and expertise of people belonging to an organization. It is a source of creativity and innovation, and therefore of the competitive advantage of an organization. (Definitions of human capital on the Web, 2005). In considering the concept of human capital increasing importance has now been given by theorists and analysts to the role of human learning within organizations and communities (OECD 2005). Closely linked to the idea of learning or capital in organizations is the notion of social capital, which has gained importance among analysts in the current decade. Social capital refers to the components of social life, namely, the existence of networks, policies, institutions, relationships and norms. These aspects of social life enable people to act together, create synergies and build partnerships (OECD 2005). There is complementarity between human and social capital. Social capital can influence the ability to acquire human capital through, for example, the enhancement of learning at school by strong communities (OECD 2005).

Goodland and Daly (1996) argue that social capital requires the maintenance and replenishment of shared values by communities, social and religious groups. Also, it has been suggested (OECD 2005) that in order to preserve social capital for sustained economic growth and development it is necessary to foster networks of trust and knowledge creation and sharing at the organizational, community and regional as well as between different sectors, such as government, higher education and business.

As indicated, within the wider health sector, sustainability has become synonymous with self-sufficiency in financing and often applied to situations where external aid agencies sought to induce developing country governments to take on the responsibility for funding activities that previously had been donor funded

However, as also mentioned, in immunization because of the nature of immunization and the international interest in the success of immunization programmes, the focus of sustainability has moved from this narrow meaning toward a broader concept that focuses on other aspects, such as – mobilization and allocation of adequate internal and external resources for the EPI.

Consequences of Sustainability

Many consequences of sustainability are outlined in the literature. For example, an extensive literature review (Christopher et al 2013) outlines the following important consequences and goals in the application of sustainability to healthcare including public health in recent years as seen by commentators and scholars: improvement of health, healthcare policies, or programmes; grounding healthcare policy and planning in social ecology; protecting environmental resources; maintaining the survival of healthcare organizations; continued development and fine-tuning, and targeting of programmes; institutionalization; renewability and inter-generalization equity.

Operational Definition

This includes the following:

- Continued use of programme components and activities for the continued achievement of desirable programme and population outcomes (Scheirer et al., 2011).
- Continuation, confirmation, maintenance, durability, continuance, and

institutionalization (the continued use of programme components and activities beyond their initial funding period and sometimes to continuation of desired intended outcomes (terms and their usual meaning used by researchers cited by Scheirer et al 2011).

- Alignment, compatibility, or convergence of (1) problem recognition in the external organizational environment or community (2), the program in question and (3), internal organizational objectives and capacities (Yin et al 1977; Altman 1995; Gruen 2008; Katz 1963)

The meaning of these positions is a multilevel system of a health programme implemented by individuals, internalized in an organization, functioning within a community context or inter-organizational network over time (Katz 1963). Therefore, research on sustainability which the following section deals with can require several layers of data collection to capture the multiple components of the systems involved in such continuation (Scheirer et al, 2011) This is demonstrated by the SIA framework (Chapter 6) and the case study which exemplifies it (Chapters 7-10). These emphasize a multi-method approach to gathering data on influences of programme sustainability from various sources and levels.

Sustainability Assessment

Some writers (e.g. Christopher et al, 2013) have suggested that because of the lack of any agreed-upon definition of sustainability, as already mentioned, it simply has not been possible for healthcare researchers to evaluate empirically the outcomes of applying policies based on diverse conceptualizations of sustainability. However, they say that sustainability has been used as a central yardstick for guiding healthcare policy and planning and efforts have been made to operationalize and develop measures for it, such as indicators, benchmarks, auditing and accounting procedures, assessment protocols, and various types of reporting systems. Christopher et al (2013) also suggest that these procedures are still evolving, and there are no universally agreed upon protocols. Box 14 presents examples of methodological approaches and limitations reported in studies assessing sustainability in public health drawn from the literature (eg. Stirman et al 2012; LaPelle et al 2006; Schell et al 2013; Scheirer 2011).

Box 14: Examples of methodological approaches/elements reported in studies assessing sustainability in public health

Area of Study

- Sustainability or its influence on health programmes
- Community health programmes emphasized by studies, mostly programmes on disease prevention
- Fidelity/integrity of an intervention/practice
- Post- implementation of an intervention, programme, etc
- Continued service delivery or combination of multiple activities
- Target intervention and supporting organizational processes
- Programmes after defunding
- Factors and strategies facilitating or inhibiting programme sustainability

Design/Approach

- Mostly or solely quantitative approaches used
- Relatively less qualitative approaches used
- Both quantitative and qualitative approaches used
- Mostly naturalistic rather than experimental designs used

Unit of Analysis

- Mostly multiple implementation sites or settings, followed by individual or private level
- Single systems or communities, at a single site, among individual providers within sites, or at the team level

Timeframe

- Mostly two years or more post-implementation
- Twelve months or less post-implementation

Terms & Definitions

- The term "sustainability" is used mostly in studies
- Mostly studies did not include a working definition or model of sustainability
- Sustainability defined differently in studies
- Definitions most commonly generated by the researcher
- Definitions refer to continuation of an innovation within an organization or community

- Operational definitions frequently cited Scheirer's (2011) definition of sustainability
- Some studies were guided by a conceptual framework which included four influences or processes linked to sustainability: organizational context, influences related to the innovation, processes and capacity (internal and external)

Theory

- Grounded theory
- Institutional theory
- Organisational culture
- Diffusion of innovation
- Researchers seldom draw from theory to explain observations and test hypothesis

Methods of Data collection

- Mainly exploratory and descriptive methods
- Self-report measures
- Interviews
- Observations
- Record reviews
- Information technology systems: telephone, e-mail or Internet, etc
- Case studies combining multiple sources of data
- Less attempts at developing and testing tools for assessing sustainability

Outcomes reported

- Various outcomes reported
- Some multiple outcomes reported
- Frequently reported outcomes include proportion of providers or sites sustaining or discontinuing an innovation or programme, or the proportion of patients receiving an innovation during a follow-up period
- Also, studies frequently reported changes in the rate of programme implementation and /or recipient outcomes
- Some studies reported some form of health outcome (e.g., sustained impact or increases/decreases in desired outcomes
- Some studies fail to report sustainability outcomes or data properly

It is worth emphasizing that there are other sustainability assessments that are not related only to "environmental and ecological" type assessments. As indicated above, there are other agencies such as several US agencies, including the US Environmental Protection Agency, which does include public and individual health factors in sustainability related decisions. The US EPA Sustainability Assessment and Management Framework (EPA 2011) is an approach to incorporating sustainability to inform decision making. The steps involved in this approach are as follows:

- A screening evaluation to determine whether to conduct the Sustainability Assessment and Management process and to determine the appropriate level of effort or depth of such an assessment.
- Problem definition and scoping, which includes identification of options, preliminary scoping of the analysis, stakeholder involvement, and opportunities for collaboration.
- Use of a set of analytic tools in the Sustainability Assessment and Management process.
- Integration of the Sustainability Assessment and Management process into management and policy decisions. Integration into decision making involves summarizing the major results of the assessment in terms of a trade-off and synergy analysis that highlights impacts on important social, environmental, and economic objectives.
- Presentation of results to the decision makers.

To incorporate sustainability effectively within the EPA and to achieve external adoption in various sectors, the EPA says it will have to make use of a variety of assessment tools. EPA will need to develop a set of tools or models that can be used to quantify impacts on important, social, environmental, and economic indicators that might be affected. Box 15 presents summaries of descriptions by the EPA of selected sustainability tools. According to the EPA, this list is not intended to be a comprehensive list of potential tools but rather a brief review of some important assessment tools.

Box 15: Overview of Selected Sustainability Tools

Risk Assessment: Risk assessment is a tool widely used for characterizing the adverse human health and ecologic effects of exposures. Classically, risk assessments for human health endpoints involves four major steps: a hazard identification, dose-response assessment, exposures assessment and risk characterization.

Life-Cycle Assessment: Life-cycle assessment is a "cradle-to-grave" analysis (or "cradle-to-cradle" of environmental impacts from production, use, and eventual disposal of a product. Life-cycle assessments are used to analyze the major environmental impacts of various products, to determine how changes in processes could lower the environmental impact, and to compare the environmental impacts of different products.

Benefit-Cost Analysis: Benefit-cost analysis is a widely used tool from economics to evaluate the net benefits of alternative decisions. Benefit-cost analysis seeks to assess the change in welfare for each individual affected by a policy choice, measured in a common monetary metric, under a set of alternatives.

Ecosystem Services Valuation: Ecosystem services are goods and services that contribute to human well-being and are generated by ecosystem processes. For example, ecosystems can filter contaminants to provide clean water for human use and modulate water flow, reducing the probabilities of flooding and providing higher flows during drier periods.

Integrated Assessment Models: Integrated assessments cross disciplinary lines to merge theory and data from multiple disciplines to address complex environmental issues.

Sustainability Impact Assessment: Sustainability impact assessment is used to analyze the probable effects of a particular project or proposal on the social, environmental, and economic pillars of sustainability.

Environmental Justice Tools: Environmental justice tools are analytic methods for judging whether communities are experiencing inordinately high environmental and health burdens and for evaluating the sustainability of communities.

Present Conditions and Future Scenario Tools: The Sustainability Assessment and Management approach requires an evaluation of present and future conditions to show that present decisions and actions are not compromising future human and ecologic health and well-being.

Source: EPA (2011)

As can be seen from Box 15, the EPA Sustainability Assessment and Management Framework represents a variety of tools that provide public health researchers opportunities to assess a range of sustainability issues that have much public health policy relevance, such as change in welfare for people affected by policy change, water and sanitation and health burdens. Indeed, Sustainability Impact Assessment which is one of many sustainability assessments tools included in the US EPA Sustainability Assessment and Management Framework is used in this book to illustrate the role Sustainability Impact Assessment can play in assessment of public health policy change processes based on a case study connected to immunization policy in the Gambia. The SIA tool is described in much detail in Chapter 5.

Challenges for Sustainability implementation

Generally, there are many sustainability challenges that are raised by the cost concerned with changing to different methods of entertaining, working and living. These include people not being convinced of the need for change; people not being willing to change the way they do things; the fact that sustainability usually concentrates on long-term problems; the cost involved in changing to different methods of working, etc; the novelty and lack of related technology; and lack of government commitment. Box 16 describes these sustainability challenges in detail.

Box 16: Different types of Sustainability Challenges
There are a number of sustainability issues that prevent mass changes of behavior. To begin with, many people simply are not convinced there is a need for change. Other people view change with skepticism because the new methods are not proven, yet they require a great deal of financial investment. Furthermore, governments could serve as models in the movement toward sustainability, but many lack the commitment to do so. One of the major sustainability issues is getting mass support. People generally do not like to change simply for the sake of doing things a different way. It is often necessary, therefore, to provide a reason to shift to sustainable methods. Attempts to do this are often hindered by conflicting information. While some people are emphasizing the dire need for change, many others are arguing that sustainable solutions are being developed for problems that are overstated or non-existent. Another reason mass support is difficult to obtain is because sustainability often focuses on problems that have not occurred yet. It is generally more difficult to get people to take preventive measures than it is to get them to act on solving a current problem. That many of the concerns raised by promoters of sustainable methods address problems that will occur in the distant future only aggravate the difficulty. Even when there is adequate support, the expense involved with shifting to different methods of living, working, and entertaining raises many sustainability issues. Many of the sustainable solutions require large scale changes. For example, if a whole community was required to change to a new sustainable heating method, every level of society would be affected. This includes the individual who has to buy new heating equipment, the energy company that has to invest in new production and delivery infrastructure, and the government that must also invest and regulate the new industry. Another of the sustainability issues is the newness and lack of related technology. For people to change their methods of living, they need alternatives. In many instances, the alternatives are subjects of debate. There is little, if any, basis to believe that a given solution will work or will be as good as the previous method and many people are not willing to take the risk. Furthermore, certain problems may be recognized but there is often no technology to support a sustainable solution.

Lack of governmental commitment also presents sustainability issues. There are numerous conferences and summits held where government leaders acknowledge problems and agree upon certain proposed solutions. After those events, however, the agreements are not implemented so no real changes are made.

Source: Wise Geek (2015)

One most important challenge for the idea of sustainability concerns the different meanings ascribed to it specifically in healthcare within social development contexts. Christopher et al (2013) suggest that conceptual definitions of sustainability, although seemingly reasonable, fail to include several operational decisions that are necessary for the implementation of this ideal. As Christopher et al (2013, p 4) say:

> At a minimum, these decisions include fundamental questions of what, when, why, how, and who. Answers to the question of what is to be sustained range from population health, to healthcare policy systems, to funding levels, and to particular types of programs and treatments. Are these to be sustained for a defined period, on a con tinuous and indefinite basis, until they are shown to be ineffective, or until the need changes or better programmes and treatments are de veloped? Definitions of ideal and tolerable levels of health and dis ease inform the question of why; available technologies impact ques tions of how sustainability is sought; and moral, social, political, and spiritual values are central to answering questions of whose health is to be sustained and who should sustain it.

Christopher et al (2013) suggest that the different agendas that are provided for the ideal of sustainability and their critique is summarized by two opposing viewpoints. One is the argument by some committed ecologists that sustainability is "too human centric" (EurActiv 2006), unsupportive of nature and the many non-human species. The other is the complaint that sustainability is too "anti-progress," ... a malign philosophy...[with] low aspirations, and restraint" (Williams 2008). Christopher et al contend that such attacks on the ideal of sustainable development come from a conservative, free market perspective, arguing for the abundance of natural resources and human technological ingenuity. They outline what they see as one of the most fundamental limitations of sustainability: "the ubiquity of change, whether gradual or rapid, and the notion that states of equilibrium are the exception and that, even when they exist, they are only temporary with regular transitions between multiple equilibriums. The ongoing co-evolution of human and non-human organisms, including bacteria, as well as the constant development of new healthcare delivery systems, the discovery of more effective treatments, and the discontinuation of antiquated treatments all undermine the usefulness of sustainability as an overarching criterion or yardstick for the guiding of health care policy and planning".

Because of all these limitations, Christopher et al (2013, p.10) suggest that for the concept to have meaning, it is essential that it be more sharply delimited. One way to do this in healthcare, they say, is through focusing it on population health. But this must include the recognition that sustainability is only one of many important evaluative criteria that should inform healthcare policy and planning, such as effectiveness, efficacy, responsiveness, and equity". As will be seen in Chapter 8, the case study focused on assessing the sustainability of the expansion of the EPI and sought to, among other things, identify institutional and behavioural factors that affect the efficiency and sustainability of the EPI.

Implications for Public Health Practice and Research

The foregoing discussion suggests several implications of sustainability for public health research and practice. As mentioned, for the concept of sustainability to be meaningful it is important to delimit it more precisely by concentrating it on public health/population health (Christopher et al (2013, p). However, as also indicated, the extent to which public health initiatives are sustained is influenced by various factors and there is a need to know more about the nature of these factors and how they interwork (Stirman et al 2012). An important challenge involves assessing the barriers to and the requirements for sustaining optimal health and well-being, and this involves grappling with the difficult tradeoffs between secondary medical and rehabilitative care and interventions designed for the promotion of health, including nutrition, inoculations, sanitation, exercise, prevention of violence, and enhancing social and economic health of a population. It is population health (see chapter 1) that should be the main focus of sustainability assessments rather than specific medical treatment programmes (Stirman et al 2012).

However, while sustainability has been widely accepted as a beneficial public health/population health concept, and there is a recent increase in sustainability research, "the literature has not developed a widely used paradigm for conducting research that can accumulate into general sable findings" (Scheirer et al 2011). Box 17 presents a summary drawn from the literature of several factors (Stirman et al 2012; Scheirer et al 2011) that make it difficult to study sustainability and draw conclusions for evidence-based public health practice.

Box 17: Factors that make it difficult to study sustainability

- A fundamental challenge is the tension that exists between the continuation of interventions as originally designed and the need to adapt them for use in contexts that may differ in important ways from those in which they were originally developed and tested.
- A number of conceptualizations of sustainability have been proposed that reflect differing priorities and perspectives on this issue.
- In some models, the intervention, rather than the system into which it is introduced, is the focal point of interest.
- Such models tend to identify a set of factors or conditions that increase the likelihood of sustainability of a specific intervention.
- This approach is very different from models and studies that examine sustainability from an ecological or complex-systems perspective.
- These models emphasize the interconnection between broader environmental forces, contextual influences, and the program or intervention itself.
- The differing approaches have important implications for the way that research is conducted and the conclusions that can be drawn. For example, the former perspective may reflect an emphasis on determinants of the preservation, fidelity to, or discontinuation of a program or intervention.
- In contrast, research conducted from an ecological perspective would seek to understand the ways in which the intervention and the local context mutually adapt and evolve and how this process impacts sustainability.
- Additional challenges to the study of sustainability and interpretation of the literature include the numerous definitions and related but not entirely equivalent terms that have been used in differing fields, and variation in the timing and method of assessment employed across studies.
- Furthermore, the assessment of programs, practices, and interventions as varied as community-level prevention programs, medical records systems, psychotherapies, and quality-improvement programs will necessarily limit the extent to which assessment can be standardized.
- Data-collection methods are often constrained by relatively limited funding for follow-up research
- Another unresolved question is timing: when should data be collected to assess whether a project is sustained? Research has been conducted at a variety of time spans after focus funding ended, from 6 months to 6 or more years.

Source: Stirman et al (2012); Scheirer et al (2011)

These difficulties should serve as the basis on which public health researchers can learn by doing and improving methodological approaches that could better provide needed research evidence for improved public health practice. This principle is highlighted by the SIA framework (EU, 2003).

Summary

This chapter has offered insights into the attributes and characteristics of the term sustainability. It has offered a conceptual framework and an operational definition of sustainability as applied to public health, outlined facilitators of sustainability, its consequences and related concepts. Also, it has described sustainability assessment approaches and methods, challenges of sustainability implementation, and implications of sustainability for practice and research. All these serve to remove some of the misunderstandings about the meaning of sustainability, to show how sustainability may be usefully advanced and to harmonize discrepancies connected to misjudgments and ineffective use of the concept. As Christopher et al (2013) suggest the needs of a population's health and the application of the range of these criteria for evaluating various healthcare alternatives should be the central considerations in both sustainability assessments and, more broadly, healthcare planning. This is a principal theme in this book. Dealing with such issues has a lot to do with public health policy change which is another significant theoretical contributor to the SIA framework and the related case study and is the subject of the following chapter.

3

Public Health Policy Change

As we shall see in Chapter 6, Sustainability Impact Assessment is about assessing the impact of proposed policies and is therefore closely connected to policy change. In fact, the entire SIA process starts in the preliminary stage with a description of a proposed policy and an initial assessment of possible impacts of the policy to determine whether and to what extent an SIA is needed (OECD 2010). Policy change refers to a new direction in public policy (Bryant, 2002). As already mentioned, policy change is important to public health in two ways. The development of healthy public policy has been recognized as a cornerstone of the new public health (WHO, 1986). Also, public health programmes are developed to reflect policy aims of local departments and units. This chapter presents an analysis of policy change to determine the attributes, characteristics and other features of policy change to improve general clarity and understanding of the concept as it relates to public health. It begins with a description of the meaning of public health policy change.

Definition

"Policy" refers to laws, regulations, administrative actions, procedures, guidance, as well as incentives, or voluntary practices of governments and other institutions. Policy decisions are often shown in resource allocations. Policies in various sectors can influence health, as we have seen in the examples in Chapter 1 and a following section on the consequences of public health policy change. One example is transportation policies that can encourage physical activity. A clear health policy can define a vision for the future; it can outline priorities and the expected roles of different groups; and it can build consensus and inform people (WHO, 2011)

In public health, policy development and change incorporate advancement and implementation of public health law, regulations, or voluntary practices that influence organizational change, systems development and individual behaviour to advance improvements in health. Such policies can be implemented within the health sector, for example, a policy to expand the immunization services in The Gambia through the introduction of new vaccines, which the case study (Chapters 7-10) deals with. In addition to the health sectors, other sectors like education, agriculture, or employment can also participate in the realization of public health goals.

Thus, policy development and change is an important public health function. Policy development is included in three of the 10 Essential Public Health Functions (Box 6, Chapter 1). Public health professionals play an important role in policy development by carrying out these functions, such as conducting policy-relevant research (CDC, 2015).

Issues Preceding Public Health Policy Change

These include:

- Contentious debates about public health in countries like the United Kingdom, focusing on, for example, a ban on smoking in public places, food labeling and food advertising to children (Jachelson, 2005).
- The argument that any government intervention in these areas is an unnecessary intrusion into people's lives
- The argument that only the state can effectively reduce the poverty that is so often the root cause of ill health.
- The argument that legislation brings about changes those individuals on their own cannot, and sets new standards for the public good.
- The argument that government has a responsibility for protecting national health, and to serve in the public interest and for the public good (Saltman and Ferroussier-Davis 2000, cited by Jachelson 2005).
- The recognition that the quality and availability of health services, such as the social determinants of health (chapter 1) to populations are usually a result of public policy decisions made by governing authorities and the need to include health and health equity into all public policies as a way of enhancing collaboration between sectors and ultimately promoting health (e.g., Dahlgren et al 2006).

Characteristics of Public Health Policy Change

The characteristics of policy change have been described in the literature. For example, policy change has been identified by two patterns (Hall 1993):

- Normal, or routine, or incremental policy change- a continuation of existing policy with only slight variations from existing policy. Usually practices and policies are inclined to be a continuation of past practices and policies.
- Paradigmatic policy change- a representation of a basically new direction in state policy. It also means the simplification of the appearance of a new model or approach to thinking about a policy issue.

In public health, these two patterns of policy change occur under different political and social conditions. They can shift from focusing, for instance, on hospital and diagnostic services to health promotion and disease prevention, which has a wider focus on social, political, economic and environmental conditions, which contribute to human health. Such a change can be seen as a shift in the way of thinking on how we comprehend health and the causes of illness (Bryant, 2002).

Facilitators

The organizational, professional, and social contexts into which a policy is introduced may facilitate or block policy change. As we have seen in Chapter 1, there are multidisciplinary teams of public health workers and professionals that carry out public health functions. For example, implementation of a policy is facilitated by professionals working in hospitals and public health units, often with related but different mandates. There are governments that enact and enforce policies, such as imposing universal changes in practice standards. Also, there are social groups who are the subject of a policy that can facilitate the formulation and implementation of policy (Bryant, 2002). Policy change can involve (1) competition within the policy community and (2) competition for power and conflicting activities within the community that arise to address a policy issue (Bryant, 2002). The following are some important individuals, groups and environmental influences that can facilitate (or constrain) policy change (Sabatier 1993):

- Members of an advocacy coalition that share a set of normative and fundamental beliefs or ideology. These beliefs shape policy positions, instrumental decisions, and information sources selected to support specific policy positions. For example, in two communities along the Arizona-Mexico border, community coalitions that administered a comprehensive diabetes prevention and control intervention expanded their membership to become policy and advocacy coalitions with broad community representation. These coalitions, or Special Action Groups (SAGs), identified and prioritized policy issues that directly or indirectly affect physical activity or nutrition (Meister et al 2005).

- Several factors can influence an advocacy coalition and its activities as well as its success in achieving policy change. These include stable influences that can frame and constrain the activities of advocacy coalitions. Examples of such influences are the social, legal and resource characteristics of the society that can last for many years. They also include dynamic influences like external changes or events in global socioeconomic conditions that can change the membership and resources of various coalitions. Likewise, changes in senior level personnel within government ministries can also affect the political resources of different coalitions and their influence on decisions at the policy and operational levels.
- Enduring changes in thought or behavioural intentions that are grounded on previous policy experience. Such learning occurs through internal feedback mechanisms and includes perceptions of external dynamics and increased knowledge of problem parameters. Such learning is instrumental, as decisions about which health promotion policy model to pursue are likely to be made on purely rational grounds in relation to efficiency and effectiveness (Chapter 1).

Also, there are factors in the policymaking process that can facilitate (or inhibit) policy change, as suggested by Kingdom's (1984) and Hall's (1975) models and other ideas of policy change described in the following section.

Models of Policy change

Discussions of models of policy change are rare in the public health literature. However, the political science literature presents a range of useful and prominent policy change models and approaches (Bryant 2002). One of such models considers policy change as often occurring at the following multiple levels (Kingdom 1984):

- Upstream interventions involve policy approaches that can affect large populations through regulation, increased access, or economic incentives. For example, increasing tobacco taxes is an effective method for controlling tobacco-related diseases.
- Midstream interventions occur within organizations. For example, worksite-based programmes that increase employee access to facilities for physical activity show promise in improving health.
- Downstream interventions, which often involve individual-level behavioral approaches for prevention or disease management.

There is also the policy-making process model which Kingdom (1984) usefully illustrates as follows:

- There is forward movement of policy when elements of three "streams" come together (these "streams" are different than the upstream, midstream, and downstream metrics noted above). These three streams are (1) the definition of the problem (e.g. a high cancer rate) (2) development of potential policies to solve that problem (e.g. identification of policy measures to achieve an effective cancer control strategy) and (3) the role of politics and public opinion (e.g. interest groups supporting or opposing the policy).
- For policy change to occur there must be opening of a "window of opportunity" and the pushing of the three streams through policy change as Figure 4 illustrates.

Figure 4: Kingdom's three-stream model of agenda setting

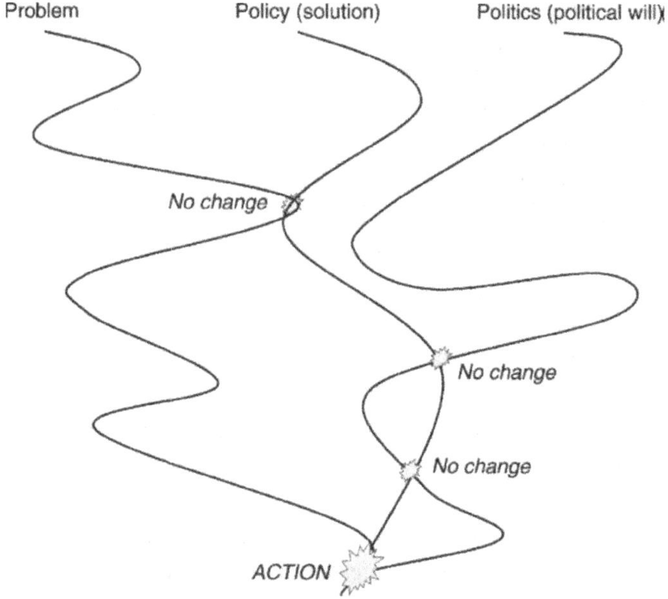

Source: Buse et al (2005), as adapted from Kingdom (1984)

Kingdom's model suggests that policy makers are at times faced with random, disjointed and disorderly data (Kingdom 1984). Thus, public health practitioners and researchers need to engage in metrics identification for assessing burden, priority setting, and measurement of progress. This will help in decision making and improvement, expansion, or termination of policies (Bryant,

2002).

Bryant (2002) suggests that Sabatier's (1993) (discussed under the "Facilitators" section above) and Hall's (1993) (discussed under the "Characteristics of public health policy change" section) policy change approaches would be of much interest to health promotion (a component of public health) as they consider the role of knowledge, ideas and learning as key elements in the process (Hall, 1993; Sabatier, 1993). As Bryant (2002, p3) says, "health promotion is an approach that stresses new ways of thinking about means to improve well-being. Analysis of models that consider how some ideas is accepted and others rejected should provide insights into health promotion's successes and failures in influencing policy development".

Another widely used and notable model is Hall's model (Hall et al 1975) described in box 18.

Box 18: The Hall model: legitimacy, feasibility and support

This approach proposes that only when an issue and likely response are high in terms of their *legitimacy, feasibility* and *support* do they get onto a government agenda. Hall and her colleagues provided a simple, quick-to-apply model for analyzing which issues might be taken up by governments (Hall et al. 1975).

Legitimacy

Legitimacy is a characteristic of issues with which governments believe they should be concerned and in which they have a right or even obligation to intervene. At the high end, most citizens in most societies in the past and the present would expect the government to keep law and order and to defend the country from attack. These would be widely accepted as highly legitimate state activities.

Feasibility

Feasibility refers to the potential for implementing the policy. It is defined by prevailing technical and theoretical knowledge, resources, availability of skilled staff, administrative capability and existence of the necessary infrastructure of government. There may be technological, financial or workforce limitations that suggest that a particular policy may be impossible to implement, regardless of how legitimate it is seen to be.

Support

Finally, support refers to the elusive but important issue of public support for government, at least in relation to the issue in question. Clearly, more authoritarian and non-elected regimes are less dependent on popular support than democratic governments, but even dictatorships have to ensure that there is some support among key groups, such as the armed forces, for their policies. If support is lacking, or discontent with the government as a whole is high, it may be very difficult for a government to put an issue on the agenda and do anything about it (see Easton's model of the political system in Chapter 3).

Thus the logic of the Hall model is that governments will estimate whether an issue falls at the high or low end of the three continua of legitimacy, feasibility and support. If an issue has high legitimacy (government is seen as having the right to intervene), high feasibility (there are sufficient resources, personnel, infrastructure) and high support (the most important interest groups are supportive – or at least not obstructive), then the odds of the issue reaching the policy agenda and faring well subsequently are greatly increased.

Of course, this does not rule out more tactical reasons for putting an issue onto the policy agenda. Sometimes, governments will publicly state their position on a particular issue to demonstrate that they care, or to appease donors who demand a response as a condition of aid, or to confound the political opposition, even when they do not expect to be able to translate their concern into a policy that could be implemented because it has low feasibility and/or support.

Source: Buse et al (2005)

Buse et al (2005) suggest that while both crisis and politics-as-usual models, such as the ones we considered above, are useful in helping to explain how issues get to the policy agenda and are dealt with, or why ultimately they are rejected (because they may lack legitimacy, feasibility or support or because the three policy streams do not come together in favorable circumstances to provide a 'window of opportunity'), observable actions are not sufficient enough to guide decision-making on all policies. As Buse et al (2005, p.73-4) indicate "you need to think about the possibility of non-policy making, or non-decision making when thinking about what gets onto the public policy agenda… Those with enough power are not only capable of stopping items reaching the agenda, they are also able to shape people's wishes so that only issues deemed acceptable are discussed, never mind acted on".

Buse et al (2005) give an example of non-decision making in relation to the market reforms in many health care system in the 1990s. They suggest that such market reforms that were usually radical rarely oppose the monopoly control used by the medical profession concerning who should or should not give treatment and prescribe drugs for patients. As Buse et al (2005, p.74) explain, "while many previous assumptions as to how health care systems should be managed and directed were overturned (e.g. privatization of public hospitals and competition between providers), the fundamental interests of the dominant occupational group prevented any concerted debate about opening medical work to other professions".

Readers are referred to the health policy literature, including Buse et al's (2005) work Making Health Policy for further exploration of how the main actors in the policy process, particularly the government and the media, put issues on the policy agenda. These main actors include government, the business community, the medical profession and other interest groups and the media. The media in most circumstances play a primary role in policy making of helping to set the policy agenda, not in other spheres of the policy process (Buse et al, 2005).

Related Concepts

As can be seen from the foregoing discussion, two of the many concepts that are related to policy change in public health are politics and evidence that can influence the decision of a government, private sector business or other group to adopt a specific policy. Evidence-based policy relies on the use of quantitative and qualitative study methods to identify programmes and practices aimed at improving policy relevant outcomes (Brownson et al., 2009). Usually political debates revolve around personal health care policies, particularly those that try to reform health care delivery. Such debates can typically be classified as either economic or philosophical. Philosophical debates centre on questions about three other ideas related to policy change, individual rights to health, ethics and government authority, while economic topics include yet another related concept, efficient maximization of health care delivery and costs.

The idea of social learning is also related to the concept of policy change. Hall (1993) connects the concept of policy paradigm (ideas that specify policy goals and determine the nature of problems that will be addressed in policy-making) to social learning. According to Hall, social learning can assume different forms, depending upon the type of changes in policy that are involved. For Hall, social learning emphasizes the role of ideas in policy making, a process that is dominated by officials and highly placed experts.

Consequences of Public Health Policy Change

The literature suggests that there are numerous consequences/achievements of public health policy change. The many achievements of public health outlined in Box 9, Chapter 1, were influenced by policy change. They include the 10 great public health achievements of the 20th century, such as seat belt laws or regulations governing permissible workplace exposures.

Operational Definition

Operational policies are the rules, regulations, guidelines, and administrative norms that governments use to translate national laws and policies into programmes and services (Cross, et al 2001). The policy process encompasses decisions made at a national or decentralized level (including funding decisions) that affect whether and how services are delivered. This is exemplified in the case study which showed that decision-making on EPI expenditure varies according to the level at which decisions are made, with officials of donors and Government making decisions on the use of EPI resources based on Government policy, prepared projects and budgets (usually without the involvement of providers at the periphery of health care), and donor conditions, while the use of EPI funds at the provider level, particularly at the level of the health facility, are predetermined by decisions taken at central level. Thus, attention must be paid to policies at multiple levels of the health system and over time to ensure sustainable scale-up. A supportive policy environment will facilitate the scale-up of health interventions (Hardee et al, 2012).

Assessment of Public Health Policy change

The literature provides several methodological approaches to the assessment of public health policy change. Rychetnik et al (2002), for example, give evaluation criteria that can help to determine whether the measured outcomes of an intervention (or policy) are included (a) the interests of people who might be involved in deciding on or delivering the policy and (importantly) those affected by it; (b) unanticipated as well as anticipated effects of the policy, beneficial or otherwise; and (c) the efficiency of the policy, as well as its effectiveness.

Using these criteria one can identify the characteristics of actions that focus on, for example, environmental and policy changes to promote active living, such as the following (Litts, et al 2013):

- identified parks and recreation
- safe routes to School
- street improvements
- street scaping
- transit and parking-related projects
- infill and redevelopment-related projects

Box 19 presents examples; (Bryant 2002; Bronson et al 2010; Swerissen et al 2014) of methodological approaches/elements that are included in articles on assessment of public health policy change.

Box 19: Examples of methodological approaches/elements to assessing public health policy change

Types of policies examined by articles

- A mixture of both "big P" policy studies (eg. formal laws, rules, regulations enacted by elected officials) and "small p" policy research (eg. organizational guidelines, internal agency decisions or memoranda, social norms guiding behaviour.

Category of Articles

- Child health; maternal health; HIV/AIDS; drug use prevention; tobacco control; violence control; environmental and disaster preparedness and bio security; school health; special populations; worksite health; international health; advocacy; general policy; or health care.

Topics

- Injury prevention, hearing, heart disease prevention, public health infrastructure, and rabies control
- Health disparities (eg subgroup analysis for vulnerable populations)

Design

- Most articles relied on a cross-sectional design

Type of Data

- Economic or cost data.
- Psychometric properties of the metrics.
- Data on psychometric testing

Testing

- Testing most often reported was for reliability (eg. interrater reliability), internal consistency, or key informant validation of methods

Outcomes

- When categorizing according to 3 levels of outcomes, most were downstream, followed by midstream and upstream(discussed in the above section "Models of policy change")

Criteria

- Effectiveness

Methods of Data Collection

- Document review
- In-depth interviews

Key Informants

- Policy analysts within the provincial civil service, municipal government, those who work directly for political representatives such as cabinet ministers and city councilors, and community activists and professional policy analysts engaged in the political change activities or organizations in health and housing policy.

Data Analysis

- Interviews recorded and transcribed. Themes and issues contained within the data identified.
- Data organized using concepts and categories identified in the policy change model.
- Policy change patterns identified and coded using the typology in the policy change model: normal, paradigmatic and gradual paradigmatic change.
- Testing of initial concepts and categories on emergent understandings.
- Inductive methods of analysis used to analyze notes taken during the document review and comments from the interviews used to develop addi-

Challenges for Public Health Policy Change

As with any decision-making process in public health practice, formulation of health policies is complex and, as we have seen above, depends on a variety of scientific, economic, social, and political forces. Table 1outlines examples of barriers to implementing effective public health policy that represent major challenges for public health policy change.

Table 1: Examples of Barriers to Implementing Effective Public Health Policy

Barrier	Example
Lack of value placed on prevention	Only a small percentage of the annual US health care budget is allocated to population-wide approaches.
Insufficient evidence base	The scientific evidence on effectiveness of some interventions is lacking or the evidence is changing over time.
Mismatched time horizons	Election cycles, policy processes, and research time often do not match well.
Power of vested interests	Certain unhealthy interests (e.g., tobacco, asbestos) hold disproportionate influence.
Researchers isolated from the policy process	The lack of personal contact between researchers and policymakers can lead to lack of progress, and researchers do not see it as their responsibility

	to think through the policy implications of their work.
Policymaking process can be complex and messy	Evidence-based policy occurs in complex systems and social psychology suggests that decision-makers often rely on habit, stereotypes, and cultural norms for the vast majority of decisions.
Individuals in any one discipline may not understand the policymaking process as a	Transdisciplinary approaches are more likely to bring all of the necessary skills to the table.
Practitioners lack the skills to influence evidence-based policy	Much of the formal training in public health (e.g., masters of public health training) contains insufficient emphasis on policy-related competencies.

Source: Brownson et al (2009)

Although the above information is drawn from the US, it has much global relevance. Many developing and developed countries are facing similar constraints in efforts at developing and implementing effective public health policy change. This is illustrated by the case study (described in chapters 7-10) that exemplifies the role of the Sustainability Impact Approach.

Implications for practice and research

There are many implications of public health policy change for practice and research, many of which have already been mentioned. For example, as indicated policy development and change are included in three of the 10 Essential Public Health Functions (Box 6, chapter 1) and public health professionals play an important role in policy development by carrying out these services, including conducting policy-relevant research to improve public health practice (CDC 2015). However, as we have seen in the previous section, there are also many factors that limit the effects of such research on public health practice. These include:

- Considerable gap between what research shows is effective and the policies that are enacted and enforced.
- Often there are broad definitions of policy, including laws, regulations, and judicial decrees as well as agency guidelines and budget priorities
- The extended process of communication and interaction that is required

for research to influence policy development and change.

- The nature of scientific information, which is often vast, uneven in quality, and inaccessible to policymakers that makes the research–policy interface more complex
- Though using research-derived evidence may be a major character of most policy models, it is uncertain whether scientific evidence will carry as much weight in the real policy process environments as other types of evidence, such as policymakers' values and competing sources of information, including anecdotes and personal experience. These other factors ultimately influence public health policy (Brownson et al 2009).

Box 20 summarizes the relationship between research and health policy that suggest several implications of policy change for research and public health practice.

Box 20: A Summary of the Relationship between Research and Policy

Researchers and research are only one among a wide variety of influences on policy processes. Yet, there is no doubt that the policy making process is influenced by research: research can help define a phenomenon as a policy problem potentially worthy of attention and research provides 'enlightenment' with many ideas affecting policy makers indirectly and over long periods of time. This is facilitated by the links between policy makers and researchers, the role of the media, timing and how the research is communicated. There are also many impediments to research being acted upon, including political and ideological factors, policy uncertainty, uncertainty about scientific findings, the perceived utility of research and how easy it is to communicate. There is considerable enthusiasm at present for using a variety of brokerage and knowledge exchange mechanisms to improve the productivity of the relationship between researchers and policy makers.

The idea that researchers and policy makers comprise two culturally distinct 'communities' is potentially misleading. Neither group is homogeneous and there are areas of common ground shared by some researchers and some policy makers. Sub-sets of researchers and policy makers participate together in competing 'advocacy coalitions' or 'policy networks' around issues. This perspective suggests that research enters policy as much through influencing political argument as through the transmission of knowledge. This indicates that recent efforts to use techniques of 'linkage' and 'exchange' to bridge the supposed 'gap' between research and policy are unlikely to succeed as much as their proponents would like.

Source: Buse et al (2005)

As mentioned, in keeping with the SIA guidelines, public health practitioners should learn by doing with a view to improving research methodological approaches. They should reflect on how to enhance current approaches and to adapt it to specific policy research projects.

Summary

This chapter has considered the definition of public health policy change, issues preceding public health policy change, characteristics of public health policy change, facilitators, models, related concepts, consequences, operational definition, assessment of public health policy change, challenges, and implications for public health practice and research. Policy has had, and will continue to have, a vast impact on our daily lives and on public health indicators in part because of its long-term effects and relative low cost (Brownson et al 2009). Many of the public health programmes now being implemented have a significant focus on policy change. To improve these programmes and to further evidence-based policy, we need to use the best available evidence and expand the role of researchers and practitioners to communicate evidence gathered properly for different policy audiences to:

- understand and engage all three streams (problem, policy, politics) to implement an evidence-based policy process;
- develop content based on specific policy elements that are most likely to be effective; and
- document outcomes to improve, expand, or terminate policy (Brownson et al 2009).

Many of these policy audiences are stakeholders who have something to gain or lose through the outcome of public health policy change. Thus, their identification and management is crucial in the public health policy process, and it is to a technique used for achieving these ends, Stakeholder Analysis, the discussion in the following chapter will now turn.

4

Stakeholder Analysis Framework

As we shall see in Chapter 6, under step 4 of the SIA framework, Ensuring stakeholder participation, SIA includes, among other things, checking assumptions and assessments from the different viewpoints of various interest groups which lead to mutual understanding and more robust and justified conclusions. This also increases the acceptance and credibility of the results of the impact assessments, which should be broadly backed by the stakeholders involved. There is in all chapters of the book this recurring theme of the importance of stakeholder involvement and participation in health policy development. Stakeholders can be defined as 'organizations and individuals that are involved in a specific activity because they participate in producing, consuming, managing, regulating, or evaluating the activity'. Taking into account stakeholder perspectives, varying from an individual residing within a community to national governments to global organizations, allows health interventions to be seen from multiple angles. This has several advantages: (1) understanding the perspective of key decision makers provides information on the likelihood of policy changes required for intervention implementation, (2) consumer ideas, concerns and expectations related to the intervention can predict the likelihood of successful intervention implementation, (3) understanding multiple stakeholder perspectives allows intervention refinement incorporating innovative ideas and strategies to influence key stakeholders can be formulated, and (4) sharing perspectives between key stakeholders may enhance solidarity around a particular intervention (Hyder et al 2009). As we shall see, these suggestions are consistent with the goals of the sustainability impact assessment (SIA) approach discussed in Chapter 6, and the case study on assessing the sustainability of immunization programmes described in Chapters 7-10. The SIA approach emphasizes the participation of stakeholders on the ground that it "ensures input on the possible impacts (direct or indirect) and trade-offs from different perspectives and disciplines. This increases awareness of the wider implications of policies and the range of issues affected, and counterbalances the methodological limits to monetizing impacts" (OECD 2010, p.4). Techniques for stakeholder engagement and involvement are many and varied and can be chosen to suit a specific decision but need to address the barriers and challenges identified for each stakeholder group (Markwell 2010). This chapter deals with the stakeholder analysis technique which is another main contributor to the SIA framework and the case study. Stakeholder Analysis is a technique used to identify and assess the influence and importance of key people, groups of people, or organizations that may significantly impact the success of an activity or project (Friedman and Miles 2006). The chapter begins with a look at the historical development of the stakeholder analysis technique or framework

Historical Development

The roots of stakeholder analysis are in the political and policy sciences and in management theory where it has evolved into a systematic tool with clearly defined steps and applications for scanning the current and future organizational environment (Brugha et al 2000). The stakeholder analysis technique was used in the early 1930s in the US within strategic management in the private sector to include all the groups who had an interest in the business (Winstanley et al 1997). Here, the rationale for paying attention to stakeholders is that they are in a position to influence the wellbeing of an organization or the achievement of its objectives.

In health management, stakeholder analysis has usually been associated with organizations trying to achieve particular goals and advantages in its relationships with other organizations, by identifying potential allies and building alliances or reducing potential threats (Blair 1996). However, it appears from the literature review of the case study (Sarr, 2005) described in Chapters 7-10 that there was relatively less use of the approach in health care in general and in the EPI in particular, despite the framework being applied successfully for many years in the area of management.

Furthermore, during the past ten years in industrialized societies the focus of health policy research has changed from a retrospective analysis of the processes of health policy analysis in various environments to a relatively more systematic and less intuitive, structured and prospective stakeholder analysis carried out by organizations and development managers (Varvasovszky et al 1998). This important methodological difference between stakeholder analysis and the conventional methods of health policy analysis makes this case study significant. Also, the case study is prominent because, as mentioned, the involvement of stakeholder improves the relevance and quality of the research and increases the use of results (Burton 1999). By increasing the utilization of results the lessons learnt could be used to further develop and re–organise immunization programmes. In the case study, as in the following sections, policy actors are considered as interest groups, as well as active or passive players (persons or organizations) on the policy scene that might be related to or affected by the health policy.

Process of Engaging Stakeholders

Markwell (2010) describes the following four useful stages to support the stakeholder analysis technique to help identify which individuals or organizations to include in a policy process, project, programme, etc.

1. Identifying and mapping external and internal stakeholders (and partnerships)

The beginning of any stakeholder engagement process is stakeholder map ping, the purpose of which is to identify the target groups and pulls together as much information as possible concerning stakeholders. As already mentioned, Stakeholders' are by definition people who have a 'stake' in a situation. Stakeholders can be described in organization terms as, those who are 'internal' (e.g. employees and management) and those 'external' (e.g. customers, competitors, suppliers etc.) (Markwell 2010).

However, within the field of public health the development of strategies, programmes and projects may well be undertaken on a cross-boundary, interdisciplinary way. For example, a local health and wellbeing strategy may be developed by (Markwell 2010):

- Internal stakeholders who participate in the coordination, funding, resourcing and publication of the strategy from a local health and well-being partnership, the local Primary Care Trust and the local authority;
- External stakeholders who are engaged in contributing their views and experiences in addressing the issues that are important to them as patients, service users, care-givers and members of the local community (Markwell 2010).

The questions in box 21 (Markwell 2010) are designed to reveal the stakes as well as help to identify the right people to involve in any particular situation.

Box 21: Questions to reveal the stakes as well as help to identify the right people to involve in any particular situation.
• Who is or will be affected, positively or negatively, by what you are doing or proposing to do? • Who holds official positions relevant to what you are doing? • Who runs organizations with relevant interests? • Who has been involved in any similar situations in the past • Whose names come up regularly when you are discussing this subject?

Table 2 (Markwell, 2010) presents examples of internal and external stakeholders based on a Public Health Department within a Primary Care Trust.

Table 2: Internal and External stakeholders

Internal Stakeholders	External Stakeholders
• Director of Public Health • Head of Health Intelligence and Information • Procurement • Director of Nursing • Public Health Strategists • Public Health Management Analyst • Director of Programmes and Services • Research Scientist • Communications • Environmental Health Intelligence Analyst • Public Health Manager • Trustees • Board committee members	• Local Authority/council • Providers • Acute trusts • Patients • Service users • Customers • Suppliers • Funders • Quality assessors • LINk group (the largest provider of services in Australia's superannuation fund administration industry, which services the fourth largest pension pool in the world based on funds under management) • Special interest groups • Health visitors/school nurses • Wider public health workforce • Media

Source: Markwell (2010)

Identification of stakeholders may depend on where people work. For example, those who work in a commissioning organization rather than in an organization that provides services should recognize the organizations that provide services as an important group of their stakeholders that include patients and service users. This is because provider organizations will be more important than competitors (Markwell 2010)

Schiller et al (2013) suggest that although a rich body of literature surrounds stakeholder theory, a systematic process for identifying health stakeholders in practice does not exist. They therefore present a framework of stakeholders related to older adult mobility and the built environment, and further outlines a process for systematically identifying stakeholders that can be applied in other health contexts, with a particular emphasis on concept mapping research. The framework consists of a three-step, iterative creation process:

- identifying stakeholder categories,
- identifying specific stakeholder groups
- soliciting feedback from expert informants.

The result of this process was a stakeholder framework comprised of seven categories with detailed sub-groups. The main categories of stakeholders are shown in Box 22.

Box 22: Main categories of stakeholders
• The Public, • Policy makers and governments • Research community • Practitioners and professionals • Health and social service providers • Civil society organizations, and • Private business.

Source: Schiller et al (2013)

A section in Chapter 9 on the case study methodology of developing and applying the stakeholder analysis tool describes how the stakeholders that included many of the categories listed above were selected.

2. Assessing the nature of each stakeholder's influence and importance

This involves estimating stakeholder's influence and importance always in relation to the objectives one is seeking to achieve (Influence means simply how powerful a stakeholder is in terms of influencing direction of the project and outcomes. Importance simply implies those stakeholders whose problems, needs and interests are priority for an organization). For the purpose of achieving programme or project success it is necessary to assess effectively these important stakeholders (Markwell 2010). Box 23 presents some examples of types of direct and indirect influences (Markwell 2010).

Box 23: Examples of types of direct and indirect influences

Direct influence

- legal hierarchy (command control of budgets)
- authority of leadership (charismatic, political)
- control of strategic resources (suppliers of services or other inputs)
- possession of specialist knowledge
- negotiation position (strength in relation to other stakeholders)

Indirect Influence

- social, economic or political in status
- varying degrees of organization and consensus in groups
- ability to influence the control of strategic resources significant to the project
- informal influence through links with other groups other stakeholders in

Table 3 below identifies both the sources and indicators of influence that internal and external stakeholders may hold.

Table 3: Stakeholder Sources of Influence

Internal Stakeholders	External Stakeholders
• Hierarchy (formal power) e.g. authority, senior position • Influence (informal power) e.g. leadership style • Control of strategic resources e.g. responsibility for strategic products • Possession of knowledge and skills e.g. expert knowledge that forms the organizations core competence	• Control of strategic resources e.g. materials, labour, money • Involvement in strategy Implementation e.g. strategic partners in distribution channels • Possession of knowledge and skills e.g. cooperation partners, subcontractors • Through internal links e.g. networking

• Control of the environment e.g. negotiation & network of relationships to external stakeholders • Involvement in strategy implementation e.g. as a change agent or responsibility for strategic projects	

Source: Markwell (2010)

Different stakeholders may share the same aims in general, such as providing quality of services' or 'improving the quality of life for the community. However, if the level at which stakeholders are involved is particular they may desire to impose various aims and priorities on an organization. There is also the influence of the level of importance provided by an organization to the stakeholders' needs and interests which is also central to the success of strategy and project development. Such sources of importance can affect both internal and external stakeholders (Markwell 2010). Table 4 outlines stakeholder sources of importance.

Table 4: Stakeholder Sources of Importance

Internal Stakeholders	**External Stakeholders**
• Which problems affecting which stakeholders, does the strategy/project seek to address or alleviate?	
• For which stakeholders does the strategy/project place a priority on meeting their needs, interests and expectations?	
• Which stakeholders' interests converge most closely with the strategy/ project objectives?	

Source: (Markwell 2010)

3. Constructing a matrix to identifying stakeholder influence and importance

This involves constructing and using the influence/importance matrix (Figure 5) as a stakeholder analysis tool to identify stakeholder influence and importance (This technique can be used in relation to a particular strategic development initiative or activity, such as the launch or withdrawal of a service).

Figure 5: Influence/Importance Matrix

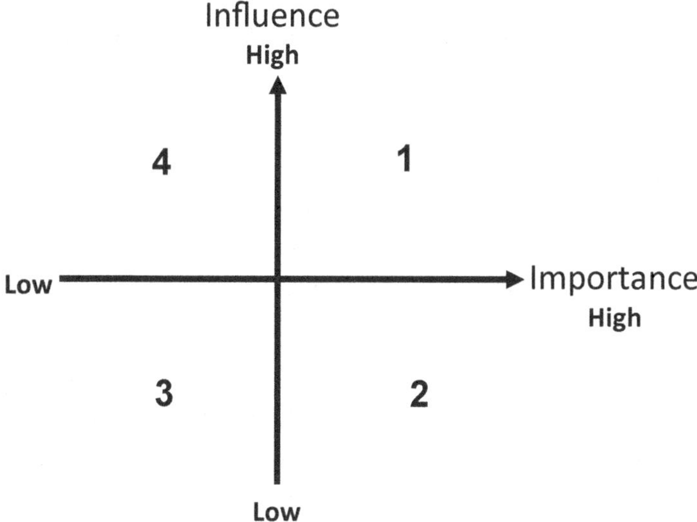

Source: Markwell (2010)

In using the tool one should first plot stakeholders in relation to how they would line up. This is the level and characteristic (for or against) of their importance and the degree of their influence. One can also plot a second map to show how one would need stakeholders to line up if the development were going to have a good chance of success.

One can compare the two maps to identify mismatches and establishing priorities for managing stakeholders. Also priorities for maintaining stakeholders in their current positioning can be established (Markwell 2010). Box 24 shows how each quadrant can be analysed in a clockwise rotation:

Box 24: Analysing each quadrant Influence/Importance Matrix

Quadrant one: Key stakeholders placed here have high influence and high importance need to be fully engaged on the strategy/project. The style of participation for stakeholders needs to be appropriate for gaining and maintaining their ownership.

Quadrant two: Stakeholders placed here can be highly important but having low influence or direct power, however need to be kept informed through appropriate education and communication.

Quadrant three: Stakeholders here have low influence and low importance and care should be taken to avoid the dangers of unfavourable lobbying and therefore should be closely monitored and kept on board.

Quadrant four: Stakeholders placed here can hold potentially high influence but low importance should be kept satisfied with appropriate approval and perhaps bought in as patrons or supporters.

However, it is important to recognise, that the map is not static, Changing events can mean that stakeholders can move around the map with consequent changes to the list of the most influential stakeholders.

Chapter 9 on the case study methodology of developing and applying the stakeholder analysis tool also outlines a process of assessing the importance, influence and positions of the stakeholders identified in stage one on the issue of whether to use the limited resources to introduce new vaccines in to the weak EPI infrastructure, or use such resources to improve the infrastructure and funding. This process was aided by the development and analysis of a stakeholder table (Chapter 9, Table 9) similar to the steps outlined above.

4. Monitoring and managing stakeholder relationships

Table 5 provides a list of principles that summarizes the key features of stakeholder management (The Clarkson Centre for Business Ethics (in Friedman and Miles (2006, p151), as cited by Markwell (2010).

Table 5: Principles of Stakeholder Management

Principle 1	Managers should acknowledge and actively monitor the concerns of all legitimate stakeholders, and should take their interests appropriately into account in decision-making and operations.
Principle 2	Managers should listen to and openly communicate with stakeholders about their respective concerns and contributions, and about the risks that they assume because of their involvement with the corporation.
Principle 3	Managers should adopt processes and modes of behavior that are sensitive to the concerns and capabilities of each stakeholder constituency.
Principle 4	Managers should recognize the interdependence of efforts and rewards among stakeholders, and should attempt to achieve a fair distribution of the benefits and burdens of corporate activity among them, taking into account their respective risks and vulnerabilities.
Principle 5	Managers should work cooperatively with other entities, both public and private, to insure that risks and harms arising from corporate activities are minimised and, where they cannot be avoided, appropriately compensated.
Principle 6	Managers should avoid altogether activities that might jeopardize inalienable human rights (e.g., the right to life) or give rise to risks which, if clearly understood, would be patently unacceptable to relevant stakeholders.
Principle 7	Managers should acknowledge the potential conflicts between (a) their own role as corporate stakeholders, and (b) their legal and moral responsibilities for the interests of stakeholders, and should address such conflicts through open communication, appropriate reporting and incentive systems and, where necessary, third party review.

Source: Markwell (2010)

Friedman and Miles (2006), as cited by Markwell (2010), have developed a stakeholder management model (Table 6) that can be used to identify the style of stakeholder management needed contingent upon Arnstein's ladder of participation. Markwell (2010) suggests that this model can be used to identify the style of stakeholder management. This model comprises twelve distinct levels (Friedman and Miles 2006) which are summarized as follows:

Highest levels-involvement, collaboration, partnership, delegated power, stakeholder control- are characterized by active or responsive attempts at empowering stakeholders in corporate decision-making.

Middle levels: explaining, placation, consultation, negotiation- stakeholders have the opportunity to voice their concerns prior to a decision being made, but with no assurance that their concerns will impact on the end result.

Lower levels: manipulation, therapy, informing- organization is merely informing stakeholders about decisions that have already taken place, although these levels represent bad practice if done in isolation.
Table 6: Style of Stakeholder Management Model

		Stakeholder Management tools and nature of response	**Intention of engagement**	**Level of Influence**	**Style of dialogue and associated examples**
Degrees of stakeholder power	Proactive or responsive/ trusting	12. Stakeholder control	Majority representation of stakeholders in decision-making process	Forming or agreeing to decisions	Multi-way dialogue e.g. community projects
		11. Delegated power	Minority representation of stakeholders in decision-making process		Multi-way dialogue e.g. board representation
		10. Partnership	Joint decision-making power over specific projects		Multi-way dialogue e.g. joint ventures
Degrees of involvement		9. Collaboration	Some decision-making power afforded to stakeholders over specific projects		Multi-way dialogue e.g. strategic alliances
		8. Involvement	Stakeholders provide conditional support; If conditions are not met support is removed. The organization decides the extent of the conformity		
		7. Negotiation		Having an Influence on decisions	Multi-way dialogue e.g. constructive dialogue
Degrees of tokenism	Responsive/ neutral	6. Consultation	Organisation has the right to decide. Stakeholders can advise. Appease the stakeholder	Being heard before a decision	Multi-way dialogue e.g. reactive bargaining
		5. Placation	Stakeholders can hear and be heard but have no assurance of being heeded by the organization		Two-way dialogue e.g. questionnaire, interviews, focus groups, task forces, advisory panels
		4. Explaining	Educate stakeholders	Knowledge about decisions	Two-way dialogue e.g. workshops
Non-participation	Autocratic/ cynical	3. Informing			One-way dialogue e.g. verified corporate reports
		2. Therapy	'Cure' stakeholders of their ignorance and preconceived beliefs		One-way dialogue, e.g. briefing sessions, leaflets, magazines, newsletters, corporate reports other publications
		1. Manipulation	'Misleading' stakeholders attempting to change stakeholder expectations		

As Markwell (2010 explains, it is likely that various stakeholder groups and the same stakeholder groups at various times will be treated at different levels and these can be affected by (1) stakeholder characteristics (2) different stages in an organization's life cycle (3) different strategies pursued by stakeholders and (4), the different focus and stage of the policy, programme, etc.

Limitations

As already mentioned, policy development is a complex process which frequently takes place in a changeable and quickly unstable context, subject to uncertain internal and external factors. As a cross-sectional view of an evolving picture, the use of stakeholder analysis for foreseeing and managing the future is time-limited and it should be correlated by other policy analysis approaches (Brugha et al 2000). The case study therefore used an integrated approach to assessing immunization systems that consists of not only of a stakeholder analysis tool that includes indicators of financial sustainability of immunization programmes, but also a complementary resource map tool that is suited to this specific application area, together with data from the EPI, government and donor records, and several interview and data collection approaches. The need for such an approach is highlighted by the SIA approach and in the relevant literature.

Summary

This chapter has described the stakeholder analysis framework, including its historical development, steps and limitations. Using the stakeholder analysis technique, policy-makers and planners of public health programmes, including immunization programmes in developing countries in particular, can identify groups that will be affected by proposed activities, their reactions to prospective changes and the roles they might play in assisting or blocking them. With this information in hand, planners can develop strategies for involving relevant central and local officials and communities, including users of the service, in reform. It is important to focus also on the users of the service as their attitudes and beliefs influence their demand for services, which in turn influences the sustainability of programmes. If roadblocks to consensus loom too large, funding can be postponed-or cancelled-until conditions for success can be achieved. This information can then be used to develop strategies for managing these stakeholders where there are broad disagreements, to facilitate the implementation of specific decisions or organizational objectives, or to understand the policy context and assess the feasibility of future policy directions such as estimating the current level of total financing for the EPI and the prospects for increasing funding through mobilisation of local and external funding; estimating the allocation of spending to priority EPI programmes and population groups, and assessing the financial importance of key players in the EPI as a guide to the development of reform strategies. The development and application of the resource map tool that complements the stakeholder analysis framework in the case study was based on the National Health Accounts methodology which is also included in the SIA framework (EU 2003) and is another significant contributor to the case study. The following chapter deals with the National Health Accounts methodology.

5

National Health Accounts Framework

We shall also see under step 5 of the SIA approach Analyzing the Economic, Environmental and Social Impact of Policy that there is a crucial need in SIA of basing the development of criteria and indicators on the capital approach, in which total national wealth is broadly defined to include: (i) financial capital such as stocks, bonds and currency deposits; (ii) produced capital such as machinery, buildings, telecommunications and other types of infrastructure; (iii) natural capital in the form of natural resources, land and ecosystems; (iv) human capital in the form of an educated and healthy workforce; and (v) social capital such as functioning social networks and institutions. These indicators or criteria are either linked to foundational wellbeing, which is essential to society, or to economic wellbeing, which is derived from market activity. Indeed, National Health Accounts (or NHAs) is a major theme for the economic pillar of the SIA. Therefore, the principles of National Health Accounts are in many ways consistent with the methodologies of the SIA and the case study. NHA is a tool specifically designed to inform the health policy process, including policy design and implementation, policy dialogue, and the monitoring and evaluation of health care interventions. First, the chapter briefly describes the NHA concept. It outlines the historical development of the concept of NHA. It outlines issues preceding NHAs, as well as the goal and utility of NHAs. It describes the role of national and international facilitators of NHAs.

It outlines the structure of the NHA framework. Finally the chapter presents limitations of the NHA concept.

Description of the NHA Concept

The NHA framework is usually defined in the literature (e.g. The Institute of Health Systems 2009 p?) as "an internationally accepted methodology used to determine a nation's total health expenditure patterns, including public, private, and donor spending". It is mainly for this reason that NHAs are used to collect expenditure data. It consists essentially of a standard set of tables that organizes, tabulates, and presents health expenditure information in a simple format. It is straightforward and policy-makers, including those without an economics or accounting background, can easily comprehend it. In addition to determining how much each of the financing sources spends on health, NHA traces the flow of resources invested and used in providing healthcare. Some important questions NHA asks are presented in Box 25.

Box 25: Some important questions NHA asked
• How are resources mobilized and managed for the health system? • Who pays and how much is paid for health care? • What goods and services are provided and by whom? • How are health care funds distributed across the different services, interventions and activities that the health system produces? • Who benefits from health care expenditure?

Source: The Institute of Health Systems (2009)

Brief Historical Development of NHA

This includes (The Institute of Health Systems 2009)

- The NHA framework adopting its fundamental principles of health accounting from the System of Health Accounts (SHA) of the Organization for Economic Cooperation and Development (OECD).
- The SHA giving the International Classification for Health Accounts (ICHA). The ICHA classifying health care entities and categorizes each type of health expenditure.
- Presentation of an SHA manual representing a milestone in the creation of an international standard for NHA. However, the primary audience of the SHA was high-income countries, with certain considerations accorded particularly to developing countries (For example, OECD methodology for NHA does not clearly differentiate between financing sources and financing agents, which would be of little interest to most OECD countries where unlike developing countries governments are the source of the largest part of health care financing through general and earmarked taxation and mandatory contributions)

- The United States Agency for International Development (USAID), the World Bank (WB), and the World Health Organization (WHO), in an effort to encourage other countries to produce NHA, jointly sponsoring the development of a complementary manual, "A guide to producing National Health Accounts: with special applications for low and middle income countries" (commonly referred to as the Producers Guide).
- Adoption of a methodology in the Producers Guide that expands the SHA classification scheme to enable collection of health expenditure data in the more disaggregated fashion as required by a pluralistic health system of financing and delivery. In such a health system, providers may receive payment from more than one source and payments may be made to numerous types of recipients.

Issues Preceding National Health Accounts

NHA is preceded by several issues related to the needs for health system financing information and standardized tools to capture health financing information. These needs are based on several factors including (eg Merson et al 2006; The Institute of Health Systems 2009):

- Demographic transition, changing patterns in burden of disease, technological advances and rising expectations of people leading to increasing demands on health care systems and financial resources.
- The demand for financial data that allow the accurate estimation of financing needs and allocations, which is lacking in many developing countries.
- The crucial need to know where the funds for health care are coming from and how they are being utilized, making information about the sources and uses of funds for health a key input in deciding how public funds are best used.
- The need for standardized tools to capture health financing information.
- The need to disaggregate private health expenditure into various forms of payments (such as direct fees for service), which is rarely done.

The Goal and Usefulness of NHA as a Political Tool

As already mentioned, NHA is a tool specifically designed to inform the health policy process, including policy design and implementation, policy dialogue, and the monitoring and evaluation of health care interventions. Its primary users are health system policy-makers. The main objective of NHA is providing main pieces of needed information to policy-makers (Merson et al, 2006). This is achieved through systematic collection of data on sources, agents and uses of health funds. This way NHA can give answers to several questions, such as those shown in Box 20. The following are pointers (The Institute of Health Systems 2009) on the utility of NHAs as a policy tool:

- NHA offers an international standardization of health expenditure information.
- If implemented on a regular basis, NHA can track health expenditure trends, which is useful for health care monitoring and evaluation purposes

- NHA methodology can also be used to make financial projections of a country's health system requirements. By providing comprehensive information on total health expenditure as well as flows of financing. NHAs contribute to sustainability of health expenditure (Chapter 2)
- NHA can contribute to measuring efficiency of health expenditure (Chapter 1)
- NHA data combined with non-financial data such as demographic information, disease prevalence rates and provider utilization rates, equips policy makers to make sound policy decisions and avoid potentially adverse policy choices. Two key areas where NHA can contribute is with regards to effectiveness and equity of health expenditure (Chapter 1)
- NHA results produce other indicators relevant to policy makers such as:
  - ◊ Government health expenditures as a percent of total public expenditure-to assess priority given to health care by the government viz-a viz its other activities
  - ◊ Government health expenditures as percent of total health spending – to ascertain government's role in providing health care to its population
  - ◊ Household expenditures as a percentage of total health spending – to estimate the burden of out-of-pocket expenditures borne by households
  - ◊ External aid as a percent of total health spending –to evaluate how much the government will have to allocate in the future after the donor aid ceases.

NHA has impacted policy in the following ways (MOH&SW 2013):

- Increased government investment in health
- Elevated the status of MDG priority areas
- Informed resource allocation decisions
- Held stakeholders accountable
- Informed civil society advocacy efforts
- Fostered need for greater coordination
- Monitored progress towards spending goals
- Exposed corruption and weaknesses in health systems and enhanced transparency

NHA Facilitators

Several organizations are actively involved in the development, collection, dissemination, and analysis of NHAs, including OECD, WHO, PAHO, and Partners for Health Reform plus (PHR plus). These organizations act as facilitators for country efforts and provide technical assistance and sometimes funding. WHO, PAHO, and PHR plus have worked collaboratively in many of the almost 70 countries that have conducted NHA. In addition, WHO, PAHO, and OECD assemble, organize, and cross-check country data and make them accessible to the wider public. But perhaps the WHO is the most powerful force behind the promotion of NHAs. NHAs are becoming more standardized under guidance from the WHO (Merson et al 2006). Box 26 summarizes WHO's efforts in the promotion of NHAs

Box 26: WHO efforts in the promotion of NHAs

Since the early 1960s, the World Health Organization (WHO) has collected and analyzed health expenditure data.16WHO's goal is to promote the best possible health for all people of the world, and this data collection is an effort to assist in meeting that goal. Over the past five years, WHO has developed a systematic effort to measure resource flows in the health systems. One of the principal products of this effort has been the World Health Report, an annual publication providing selected measured ratios and levels of expenditure on health in all WHO member countries.17The report includes NHA indicators on total expenditures on health, broken down into public and private expenditures, with additional detail for selected indicators. Data on external resources are also included.

Another product of the effort is WHO's NHA Website. Newly launched in 2004, it offers technical information and support for those conducting NHA, country-specific estimates of health expenditures, and other useful information, such as the ratios available in WHO's World Health Report and the absolute values and sources of information for such macro-variables as gross domestic product, general government expenditures, and average official and international dollar exchange rates.18Other resources, most notably an NHA database, are being developed.

WHO also builds the capacity of countries to generate health expenditure information through training workshops and direct technical assistance. In addition, WHO, World Bank, USAID, and other partners worked together for three years to produce the Guide to Producing National Health Accounts: With Special Application to Low-Income and Middle-Income Countries to provide assistance to countries embarking on the task of measuring their national health expenditures (World Health Organization, World Bank, and United States Agency for International Development, 2003).

Data

WHO's World Health Report and its NHA Website provide data on all financing agents and external resources in WHO's 192 member states. The report covers 16 specific indicators, including total expenditure on health as a percentage of gross domestic product, general government expenditure on health as a percentage of total expenditure on health, prepaid and risk-pooling plans as a percentage of private-sector expenditures on health, and how these relate to exchange rates.

Source: Merson et al 2006

Structure of the NHA Framework

The NHA framework consists of matrices or two dimensional tables for organizing and tabulating health spending data. Each table or matrix acquires an analytical dimension of total health spending. While some dimensions are especially suitable for helping in the estimation of total spending, others are especially suitable for making or evaluating health policy.

In total, these matrices deal with every possible demand made of the health accounts concerning system performance (The Institution of Health Systems 2009). These matrices are described in more detail in Box 27:

Box 27: Matrices of the National Health Accounts.

(1)Financing Sources

Sources refer to the entities from which financial resources are generated for health. Health spending by sources answers the question "where does the money come from for health care?' Examples in the Indian context include: governments (state, central and local), quasi government organizations, public and private sector enterprises, government organized societies and autonomous institutions, NGOs, households, donor agencies etc

(2)Financing Agents

Financing Agents are institutions or entities that channel funds provided by financing sources and use the funds to pay for, or purchase, the activities inside the health accounts boundary. Examples are state and central ministries for health, local governments, households, NGOs, social and private insurance, private and public enterprises etc. This category sheds light on the question "who manages and organizes funds for health care?" For example, the Aarogyasri scheme of the Andhra Pradesh is positioned as an health insurance scheme managed by a trust. But in reality, it is financed by the government. Here the financing source is the government and financing agent is the Aarogyasri Trust.

(3) Providers

They are the end users or final recipients of health care funds. They are the entities which deliver health services. They include hospitals, private doctors, traditional care providers, trained birth attendants, providers of collective health services etc. This category provides information on the question "To whom does the money go?"

(4)Functions

Functions refer to the services or activities that providers deliver with their funds. Information at this level answers the question" what type of service product or activity was actually produced? Examples include curative care, preventive care, family welfare services, health care administration, medical education, research etc.

(5)Resource Costs

Resource Costs are the factors or inputs used by providers or financing agents to produce the goods and services consumed or the activities conducted in the system. They include salaries and wages; drugs, materials and supplies; service costs; interest payments, capital expenditure etc.

(6)Beneficiaries

Beneficiaries are the people who receive those health goods and services or benefit from those activities. Beneficiaries can be categorized in many different ways based on their age and sex, their socioeconomic status, their health status, and their location.

Source: The Institute of Health Systems (2009)

The NHAs tables display some aspect of health expenditure cross-tabulated by two of the dimensions. One of these dimensions can be considered as the "sources" of the funds and the other dimension as the "use" of the funds. NHA tables are named by column and row which is established in long-standing health accounts tradition and marrows the flow of resources from the sources to the use. It is possible to develop nine NHA tables that show the financial flows of funds between the different dimensions, depending on policy requirements, availability of data and funds for collection of data (The Institute of Health Systems 2009), as shown in Box 28

Box 28: Nine NHAs Tables

Health expenditure by financing agent and provider (HF X HP);
Health expenditure by provider and function (HP X HC);
Health expenditure by financing agent and function (HF X HC);
Health expenditure by financing source and financing agent (FS x HF);
Health expenditure by cost of resources;
Health expenditure by age and sex of the population;
Health expenditure by socioeconomic status of the population;
Health expenditure by health status of the population;
Health expenditure by geographic region.

Source: The Institute of Health Systems (2009)

However, countries have used four of the dimensions listed as important ones for correct estimation of total health: dimensions of sources, financing

agents or intermediaries, providers, and functions (The Institute of Health Systems 2009). A core set of four NHA tables (Chapter 10, Tables 12, 13, 14 & 15) has been adopted by the case study. The tables show the flow of funds from:
Financing Sources to financing intermediaries
Financing intermediaries to functions
Financing intermediaries to providers
Providers to functions

Limitations/Challenges of NHAs

These are several limitations of NHAs including the following (Merson et al 2006; The Institute of Health Systems 2009; Rannan-Eliya et al 1994; MOH&SW):

- Health accounts focus on the financial dimension of the health system, and NHA data cover health expenditure.
- NHAs exclude expenditures that have health effects, but whose fundamental goal is not health, for instance, housing
- NHAs do not usually cover private expenditure on traditional providers, such as herbalists
- It can be difficult to define categories of financing sources, agents and uses of funds
- The health accounts themselves do not distinguish between effective and ineffective expenditures.
- Finding data on funds spent as opposed to budgeted is a major problem in collecting data on government expenditure
- Obstacles to retrieving such data include poorly developed conceptual frameworks and methodological tools relevant to the unique situations of developing nations
- Requires information from many sources
- Necessitates participation, understanding, and ownership by all stakeholders: (including public, private, and donor)
- Requires trained team members from local institutions
- Policy purpose must be clear from the beginning
- Findings need to be analysed and presented to inform policy processes

NHAs are not the answer to all health policy questions. To answer many policy questions, NHA information must be combined with non-financial data from sources such as epidemiological studies, population surveys, and the like. Again, this need for a multi-method approach to address the limitations of

NHAs in sustainability impact assessment of policy change is highlighted by the SIA framework and the case study that illustrates the role of the SIA framework in such assessment.

Summary

This chapter has described the NHA framework in terms of its meaning, its historical development, issues that preceded its development, its goals and value as a political tool, its facilitators, and its limitations. As already mentioned, NHA is a tool specifically designed to inform the health policy process, including policy design and implementation, policy dialogue, and the monitoring and evaluation of health care interventions. Its primary users are health system policy-makers. The main objective of NHA is providing main pieces of needed information to policy-makers (Merson et al 2006). This is achieved through systematic collection of data on sources, agents and uses of health funds. This way NHA can give answers to several questions, such as how are resources mobilized and managed for the health system. However, NHAs are not the answer to all health policy questions, and must be combined with non-financial data from sources such as epidemiological studies. The significance of this is demonstrated by the SIA framework described in the following chapter, who's role in public health policy change, as indicated, this book seeks to demonstrate through the presentation of a case study in Chapters 7-10.

6

Sustainability Impact Assessment

The analyses and descriptions in Chapters 1 to 5 provide understanding of concepts and frameworks that are reflected by or are integral components of the Sustainability Impact Assessment framework. This chapter describes the Sustainability Impact Assessment (SIA) framework itself. As will be seen, SIA incorporates the concept of sustainability as a central pillar in its structures. It is an approach for exploring the combined economic, environmental and social impacts of a range of proposed policies, programmes, strategies and action plans. SIA policies, programmes, strategies, and action plans for community involve effectiveness. Such assessment can also assist decision making and strategic planning throughout the entire policy cycle (OECD 2010). This chapter aims to help enhance understanding of the fundamental components, processes and multi-dimensional nature of SIAs. It intends to increase awareness of the role of SIA for developing more sustainable policies, strategies and action plans. The chapter starts with a brief historical development of the SIA framework. It provides a general outline (OECD 2010) of what an SIA is, why it is useful, its core principles and methodologies. It sets out the steps involved in a typical SIA (OECD 2010). These are illustrated with actual examples of methodologies used in the case study outlined in Chapters 7-10. Finally, the chapter presents limitations/challenges of the SIA framework.

Brief Historical Development of SIA

Box 29 outlines the historical development of Impact Assessment (IA) which is the precursor to the SIA framework

Box 29: Brief Historical development of IA
There are many forms of IAs and no single, widely accepted approach can be detected. Starting in the 1970s, IAs were mostly used as regulatory policy appraisal in order to understand the nature of regulations and their usefulness as policy instrument as well as their impacts on businesses. These early forms developed into what is now referred to as Regulatory Impact Assessments (RIA). They are the most common forms of IA in the OECD countries. RIAs often involve environmental and social issues but their main objective is the evaluation of the costs and benefits for businesses and citizens in complying with proposed regulations. Recent examples of RIAs can be found in Ireland where in 2005 a "Report on the Introduction of Regulatory Impact Analysis" (Department of the Taoiseach, 2005) was published. A second example can be found in the UK, where in 2007 a new format for IA (previously RIA) was introduced. An IA Guidance document provides background information on practical application. Over the years, different forms of sectoral IAs have been developed, like Business Impact Assessment, Social Impact Assessment or Health Impact Assessment (Paredis et al, 2006). Methodologically, a variety of methods is used, ranging from cost-benefit analysis, multi-criteria analysis, different forms of macro- and micro-economic models, etc. Usually, quantitative assessment methods are supported by qualitative methods. In the field of environmental policy, two forms of IA have developed during the 1980s and 1990s which are seen by many as first steps towards an SIA: Environmental Impact Assessment (EIA) and Strategic Environmental Assessment (SEA).

Source: Berger (2007)

As box 23 shows, the development of SIA is widely considered to be grounded on the evolution of two kinds of IAs in the 1980s and 1990s focusing on the environment (George et al 2007), one of the three pillars of the SIA methodology. In most European countries, strategic policy management in the form of National Sustainable Development Strategies (NSDSs) became increasingly important over the last years. National Sustainability Strategies seek to integrate the three pillars of sustainability development and also supervise efforts to evaluate the implementation of the strategy objectives. It is these developments that have paved the way for the development of SIA as an integrated assessment tool (Berger 2007). The development of SIA took place originally at the Institute for Development Policy and Management, University of Manchester (University of Manchester 2014), at the initiative of the European Commission. Ex-ante assessment of policies, which is one of the main functions of SIA, has evolved since the late 1990s at a time when the EU started including social economic and environmental concerns into its policy formulation process. Ex-ante assessment, as indicated below, is a process for assessing the likely economic, social and environmental effects of policies, strategies, plans and programmes prior to them being created (OECD 2010). The SIA methodology is implemented at multi-national and national levels for EU main policy proposals. Such assessment generally includes the three complementary issues of social, economic and environmental assessment, conducted in an objective and scientific manner, and a process of consultation and dissemination among stakeholders (George et al 2007).

Main Features of SIA (OECD 2010)

- It is a methodological soft policy instrument for developing integrated policies which take full account of the three sustainable development dimensions and which include cross-cutting, intangible and long-term considerations
- It is a process for assessing the likely economic, social and environmental effects of policies, strategies, plans and programmes before they have been formulated (Ex-ante assessment)
- Sustainability in SIA means that all three sustainable development aspects are fully integrated into the assessment.
- Integrating sustainable development into policies means considering both short-term and long-term.
- It focuses beyond numbers-not allowing forms of analysis, such as cost-benefit analysis and monetization, prevail over qualitative analysis and participatory approaches.
- Participation by stakeholders ensures input on the possible impacts (direct or indirect) and trade-offs from different perspectives and disciplines, which increases awareness of the wider implications of policies and the range of issues affected, and counterbalances the methodological limits to monetizing impacts.
- It creates integrated policies which take full account of the sustainable dimensions, intangible, spatial and long-term considerations and unintended side-effects, which implies transparency and accountability at different levels
- It considers the need for matching the depth and scope of the impact as-

sessment to the significance, political and legal nature, and sectoral context of the policy proposal.

- It considers the need for establishing clear procedures on who is responsible for which steps in the SIA and the decision-making process, what methods, tools and indicators will be used, which stakeholders and experts have to be involved and in what way, and how the results will be presented and to whom.
- It requires a number of questions to be answered in the preliminary stage in order to clearly establish the nature and goals of the initiative. Box 30 presents some of these questions.

Box 30: Questions to be answered in the preliminary stage of SIA
• What is the nature and scale of the issue(s), how is it evolving, and who is most affected by it? • What are the views of the stakeholders concerned? • What are the policy objectives and what problems need to be addressed or solved? • What are the likely impacts (social, economic, ecological, and institutional) of the policy options? • What are the possible unintended (secondary) side-effects? • What changes in the target group's behaviour are desired?

Source: OECD (2010)

SIA process and steps

These consist of a closed-loop process cycle involving monitoring, adaptation and evaluation in which progress indicators are used. Although these steps suggest a logical sequence, feedback loops will also be involved because SIA is not a lineal process (OECD 2010). SIA should follow this sequence of steps (OECD 2010):

1. Screening the proposal: deciding whether an SIA is needed.
2. Scoping the assessment: deciding the extent of the assessment to be conducted.
3. Selecting tools or methodologies to match the scoping.
4. Ensuring stakeholder participation: deciding on the role of stakeholders.
5. Analysing the economic, environmental and social impacts.
6. Identifying synergies, conflicts and trade-offs across these impacts.
7. Proposing mitigating measures to optimize positive outcomes.

8. Presenting the results and options to policy makers.

These steps are described in more detail as follows:

Step1: Screening the proposal

This involves (OECD 2010):

- Determining which proposals should be examined further, which can be based on different rules, criteria or thresholds to decide those policy proposals which have characteristics or foreseeable impacts which are sufficient to trigger an SIA,
- Beginning the entire SIA process therefore with a description or definition of the initiative in question. In the preliminary stage1 an initial assessment of possible impacts, a "relevance analysis", is undertaken to determine whether and to what extent an SIA is needed.
- Using readily-available information and being more qualitative than quantitative.
- A quick scan of the potential short-term or long-term conflicts between the sustainability dimensions, for example between economic growth and environmental protection.
- Using common methods such as checklists or impact matrices are the most common methods for screening proposals.

As mentioned, the case study (Chapters 7-10) on which the methodological approach is based has assessed the sustainability of the expansion of the Expanded Programme on Immunization in The Gambia, and explored whether to use additional resources for improving efficiency in the supply chain rather than introducing new vaccines which has been the government policy. In doing this the study has considered many of the requirements, actors, phases and processes involved in such a difficult process.

The case study was conducted in the context of change in the health system in general and the EPI in particular. It coincided with the development of a financial sustainability plan for the EPI, the first of its kind in the country. As such, the study was an opportunity to let stakeholders discuss and assess their experiences and to reflect on what should be done now and in the future. Thus, the timeline for assessment of sustainability was in line with the needs of decision-makers, which is an important requirement for such assessment (Langer et al 2002)

Step 2: Scoping the Assessment

This involves (OECD 2010):

- Determining the appropriate extent and depth of the assessment, once it has been decided to conduct a sustainability impact assessment of a proposed policy.

- Matching the significance, political and legal nature, and sectoral particularities of the policy proposal to the depth and scope of the SIA, taking into account available information, time, staff and financial resources.
- Identifying the most important issues for assessment and the best ways to address them; it should set the boundaries of the impacts to be considered to ensure a focus on the most significant effects, while excluding those elements where impacts are perceived to be negligible. This can be based on the results of the screening in step one. In addition to the content of the assessment, scoping should identify the relevant criteria and indicators for sustainability adapted to the initiative, timeframe, methods, etc.
- Using similar tools for both screening and scoping (e.g. checklists, matrices, literature surveys), to reduce the time devoted to this step and helps to maintain continuity and consistency within the SIA.

In the Gambia, the period beginning 1979 when the Expanded Programme on Immunization was launched to 1994 was characterized by the following factors:

- The mobilisation of substantial resources, due to the highest priority afforded the EPI by external donors, such as the WHO, USAID, UNICEF and the Italian Government.
- During this period, the EPI has steadily increased coverage to 80% of the fully immunized child less than one year of age (Gambia EPI Review 2001).
- However, in 1994 after the coup this situation changed significantly with the progressive disengagement of many partners of the government leading to decrease in donor funding, partly due to the high priority given to the NIDs.
- The decrease in donor funding resulting in declines in immunization coverage, uncertainty of vaccine supply, aging cold chain (A cold chain or cool chain is a temperature-controlled supply chain. An unbroken cold chain is an uninterrupted series of refrigerated production, storage and distribution activities, along with associated equipment and logistics, which maintain a desired low-temperature range) equipment, interruption of outreach services due to lack of vaccines or transportation, high vaccine wastage rates, among other problems (Gambia EPI Review 2001).

These issues of instability in the EPI are therefore pertinent for this study because of their significance for the sustainability of the EPI particularly in terms of the government's ability to sufficiently finance the EPI and introduce new vaccines. The objectives (criteria) of the study are to identify appropriate tools for measuring the financial sustainability of the provision of immunization services in The Gambia, institutional and behavioural factors which affect the efficiency and sustainability of the immunization service and policy recommendations for improving or maintaining the level of immunization services in the Gambia. The study focused on indicators that the government will find useful in putting together its plan for financial sustainability under the GAVI mechanism. Unlike other indicators of financial sustainability of the EPI which have a narrower focus, the set of indicators of financial sustainability selected for the study (Levine, 2001) cover these broader, more practical aspects of financial sustainability of the EPI, as described in more detail in Chapter 8.

Step 3: Selecting tools or methodologies

This involves: (OECD 2010):

- Using several methods or tools in SIA depending on the stage of the assessment, the desired depth of scrutiny, and the specific impacts to be examined.
- Using each tool to address different issues, such as short and long-term effects.
- Matching tools selected for an SIA with the resources, capacities and timeframe available for the exercise. They should be flexible and easy to adapt to a given policy or context, and should be able to be combined so that one tool can cover areas not covered by another tool.
- Balancing qualitative and quantitative information in the different stages to achieve a sound and reliable assessment. The Sustainability A-Test (OECD 2010) presents and explains the basic instruments for performing particular tasks. This test was developed under the EU-Project to evaluate tools for sustainability assessment. The main goal was to enhance integrated assessment for sustainable development by scientifically supporting the use of assessment tools in such integrated assessment. The projected described, assessed and compared tools for this purpose. This task was aided by the application of an evaluation framework and a literature review of the use of tools and a case study to support the results. All the project results are contained in an electronic handbook called the Webbook. The Webbook gives entries for finding suitable information about tools and their support in assessment. The purpose of the Webbook is to support the selection of tools for sustainability assessment. It is available from www.Sustainability-A-Test.net (Van Herwijnen 2008). The different

categories of tools that are included in the Sustainability A-Test are shown in Box 31:

Box 31: Categories of tools that are included in the Sustainability A-Test
1. Assessment frameworks: procedural tools describing how different types of assessments are carried out (e.g. environmental impact assessment, integrated sustainability assessment). 2. Participatory tools: tools that provide broad input by stakeholders and outside experts (e.g. Delphi surveys, focus groups). 3. Scenario tools: tools that develop alternative visions of future developments or trends (e.g. trends analysis, simulations, foresight exercises). 4. Multi-criteria analysis (MCA): tools that allow joint consideration of criteria based on different measurement units (e.g. analytic hierarchy process, preference rankings, weighted summation). 5. Cost-benefit analysis (CBA): tools that assess financial and economic parameters in comparing costs and benefits (e.g. cost-benefit analysis, cost-effectiveness analysis— CBA). 6. Accounting tools: tools that present physical as well as economic and other attributes (e.g. indicator sets, measures of well-being, ecological footprints). 7. Models: tools that simulate real-world processes (e.g. general equilibrium models, demographic models, climate models).

Source: OECD 2010

According to the OECD (2010) these tools can be used in the various steps of a sustainability impact assessment, including screening and scoping (e.g. participatory tools, scenarios), impact assessment (e.g. indicator sets, cost-benefit analysis), identifying synergies and trade-offs (e.g. multi-criteria analysis), and proposing mitigating measures (e.g. modeling) The selection of assessment tools should be based on (OECD 2010):

- the stage of the assessment;
- the depth of the assessment;
- the tasks to be completed;
- the tool group most suited to the tasks; and
- the available resources.

The need for a combination of tools in SIA is shown in the case study (Chapters 7-10) which used a mixture of approaches and methods. As the SIA methodology indicates, a precondition for devising such efficient tool combinations is to know the tools which exist and the analytical results they can provide. In the case study, tools identified from the literature were assessed and reviewed with a view to selecting the most suitable tools to be used for measuring the efficiency and sustainability of the EPI, and exploring the question of whether to use additional resources for improving efficiency in the supply chain rather than introducing new vaccines which has been the government policy. This exercise lead to the development of tools and methodologies: a stakeholder analysis questionnaire, incorporating generic and country-specific indicators of financial sustainability of immunization programmes, and a resource map tool based on the National Health Accounts Methodology, together with data from the various levels of the immunization system.

Step 4: Ensuring stakeholder participation

This involves (OECD 2010):

- Involvement of a wide range of actors (not only governments).
- Making accessible the assumptions and information on which the assessment process is based
- Communicating well-founded and clearly explained decisions and outcomes.
- Open decision-making which is more effective and efficient in achieving policy results.
- Ensuring transparency and accessibility which increases stakeholder and public confidence in the policy-making process.
- Checking assumptions and assessments from the different viewpoints of various interest groups which lead to mutual understanding and more robust and justified conclusions. It also increases the acceptance and credibility of the results of impact assessments, which should be broadly backed by the stakeholders involved.
- Using participatory and qualitative exercise logic (along with quantitative measures) involving stakeholders which provides a more balanced and solid sustainability impact assessment.
- Deciding in advance for the overall SIA process the composition and representation of stakeholder groups — business, trade unions, non-governmental organizations (NGOs) and others.
- Ensuring that economic, environmental and social interests are represented.
- Determining the appropriate extent of stakeholder involvement for the specific assessment, which might include identifying the relative role of stakeholders.

- Using tools for incorporating the knowledge, ideas and inputs of stakeholders, including information technology (IT) tools to be at the core of consultations or to support the process by informing discussions. Such IT tools include electronic focus groups and participative web tools. Conventional approaches used for this purpose include consensus conferences, repertory grids technique, interactive back casting, focus groups, Delphi surveys, in-depth interviews, and scenario building exercise.
- Choosing participatory methods depending on the objectives, the content and complexity of the topics, as well as the time and resources available.

Chapter 9 describes in detail three steps (Schmeer 1999) followed in the case study to select stakeholders and ensure their participation in the stakeholder analysis:

- identification of groups and individuals relevant to immunization financing and sustainability.
- assessment of the political resources of relevant groups and individuals and their roles in the political structures to determine their relative power for the financing and sustainability of the immunization programme.
- evaluation of stakeholders' present position on the financing and sustainability of the programme, including their underlying interests and the intensity of their commitment.

Chapter 10 as well outlines in detail a three-phase process of developing and applying the resource map tool that also ensured stakeholder participation in the case study. As mentioned, this process was based on the traditional National Health Accounts (NHA) methodology. It involves:

- identification of information sources;
- data collection; and
- analysis and dissemination of results.

On the basis of the NHA methodology, a detailed inventory of public and private sector organizations and agencies involved in EPI-related activities was made. As Chapter 10 indicates, these organizations included priority stakeholders that also participated in the process of developing and using the resource map tool.

Step 5: Analysing the economic, environmental and social impacts

According to the OECD (2010) steps five, six and seven are the technical stages and constitute the "backbone" of the SIA process. For practical reasons the steps are presented in a sequence, but they are not linear, and to connect their components often feedback loops are required.

Step 5 involves (OECD 2010):

- Analysis of the short, long-term and cross-cutting economic, environmental and social effects of the proposed policy, which is the center of an SIA.
- Using baseline data that reflect the assessment objectives and criteria identified in the screening and scoping.
- Using the same types of checklist questions employed during the screening and scoping steps for identifying the most significant impacts (the analysis will however need to be more detailed and the questions specific to the sector or domain)
- Using specific sets of criteria and indicators for assessing sustainability impacts. (The use of the words criteria and indicators, however, is not always consistent. Criteria are more generic and mostly used in the ex-ante assessment process. Criteria are often formulated as questions, e.g. "Does the option affect prices consumers pay?". Indicators are more specific and mostly used for ex-post assessments and evaluations of policies and strategies, e.g., the net price difference for consumers of product type A (OECD 2010).
- Development and use of sustainability criteria to support effective policy choices, improve the quality of proposals, and reduce as much as possible uncertainties around often complex societal issues and impacts.
- Consideration of needs and consensus on purpose, scope, time investment, the existence of national sustainable development strategies (NSDS), etc in composing assessment criteria (Such choices include, among other aspects, deciding whether or not a full SIA is needed, whether an impact is significant, whether one mitigating option is better than another).
- Basing the development of criteria and indicators on the capital approach, in which total national wealth is broadly defined to include: (i) financial capital such as stocks, bonds and currency deposits; (ii) produced capital such as machinery, buildings, telecommunications and other types of infrastructure; (iii) natural capital in the form of natural resources, land and ecosystems; (iv) human capital in the form of an educated and healthy workforce; and (y) social capital such as functioning social networks and institutions. The indicators or criteria are either linked to foundational well-being, which is essential to society, or to economic wellbeing, which is derived from market activity.

The case study (Chapters 7-10) includes several sustainable criteria and indicators. These criteria that are formulated in the form of questions focusing on the particular policy area of whether to use limited resources for improving the efficiency and sustainability of the EPI, not for introducing new vaccines in the weak EPI infrastructure. Indicators were crucial to measure the sustainable outcomes, e.g. how does adding new vaccines to the EPI affect the sustainability of the EPI. In the process of developing a policy, strategy or action plan, the initial SIA criteria can evolve into concrete indicators. The case study also included both generic and country specific indicators (Chapter 8, Table 7) that cover each of the three sustainable dimensions addressed by the case study.

Thus, as suggested by impact analysis and as can be seen from the case study, using this type of indicator set could assess whether a proposed policy would contribute to the increase or decrease over time of financial, natural and social capital. Also, as indicated in the impact analysis process, this indicator framework also stresses "the need to maintain certain critical forms of capital (foundational) and the limited substitutability among different forms of capital (economic vs. foundational" (OECD 2010). The value of the indicators, as suggested is based not only on quantifying impacts but by drawing attention to important issues needing consideration

Using this approach in the case study each criterion or indicator, as indicated by the SIA framework, was given a quantitative and/or qualitative rating or score. As mentioned, a stakeholder analysis questionnaire and a resource map tool based on the NHA framework were used for the case study. Both quantitative and qualitative data analysis were conducted to gain insight into the sustainability issue the study sought to address. The aim was to help in the development of more specific and operational objectives in the country's EPI at a time when it was undergoing major reforms. According to the SIA guidelines, this approach is the foundation of the following step (identifying synergies, conflicts and trade-of(s) (OECD 2010).

Step 6: Identifying synergies, conflicts and trade-offs

This involves (OECD 2010):

- Comparing the positive and negative impacts in the different domains and to tease out potential conflicts.
- Using multi-criteria analysis to rank and compare sustainability impacts in the different pillars
- Using three basic approaches to compensate for trade-offs:
  1. A fully compensatory method allows the weak performance of one criterion to be totally compensated for by the good outcomes of another.
  2. A partial compensatory method sets limits to the ability to compensate.
  3. A non-compensatory method allows no trade-offs. In other words, "weak sustainability" allows natural or environmental capital to be

traded off against produced or manufactured capital, while "strong sustainability" does not allow for substitutions.

- Using various kinds of information expressed in different units: quantitative figures such as monetary values; physical quantities such as pollutant emissions; and more qualitative measures of human capital and social values. The measures of different types of impacts can be standardized and ranked or rated according to their perceived degree of importance.
- Considering that whatever the choice of methods, it is important to leave the final assessment of the impacts to a combination of multi-criteria analysis and democratic deliberation.

The case study provides very good examples of these approaches by posing critical sustainability questions, such as "How will the addition of new vaccines affect the sustainability of the EPI? A policy to add new vaccines in a country's EPI may have positive effects as it will help reduce the incidence of preventable diseases affecting children, such as measles, but possibly also negative impacts on EPI financing and infrastructure, especially in poor countries that are also experiencing reduction and inconsistency of donor funding. This step, which in practice is also closely linked to step seven (mitigating measures), is the most contentious for these reasons (OECD 2010): (1) Compared to economic impacts, it is usually difficult to assign monetary values to environmental and social impacts and (2) because of the difficulty of quantifying qualitative (social) aspects economic components will be given more weight in assessments and overshadow the potential ecological and social concerns, that may prove to be more important than the economic outcomes. These issues are further discussed in the final section dealing with the limitations of the SIA framework.

Step 7: Proposing mitigating measures

This involves (OECD 2010):

- Developing measures or frameworks for minimizing the potential negative effects and strengthening the positive sustainable aspects of the policy proposal (The aim is to avoid or reduce undesired impacts, while nurturing the desired impacts as much as possible).
- Using scenarios and modelling to show how mitigating measures will affect outcomes in the three dimensions.
- Giving preference to those scenarios in which none of the three sustainability dimensions is too strongly impaired.
- Ensuring that the proposed options should all meet the following minimum requirements: (j) environmental standards established to protect hu-

man and environmental health; and (ii) living standards in keeping with social well-being or to safeguard human rights. (The aim is to develop "win-win" situations where mutually- reinforcing gains can strengthen the economic base, ensure equitable living conditions, and protect and enhance the environment. Where this is impossible, the trade-offs should be clearly indicated to guide decision-makers).

- Recognizing that the importance of formulating alternatives is to move from a problem description towards concrete solutions (The advantage of this approach is that innovation and prevention are stimulated and several risks are reduced. It also has a positive effect on public participation, as different perspectives and options have been included. The possible impact on administrative burdens should be taken into account when proposing alternatives).

The case study focused as a priority on the policy to introduce new vaccines in the EPI that had already been displaying a continuous downward trend and which would be further negatively affected by the proposed policy. As suggested by the SIA framework, the case study concentrated on pertinent sustainability questions, such as whether the introduction of new vaccines will affect the sustainability of the EPI.

Also, as indicated by the SIA framework, the case study sought to identify the principal facilitating and inhibiting factors of developments in the EPI. These should include changes and additional measures to enable the three sustainable development dimensions to be better balanced.

The following mitigation hierarchy should be followed for negative effects identified in any of the domains (OECD 2010):

- first avoid, second reduce, and third offset. (Some basic rules should be respected in the appraisal process;
- for negative effects identified in any of the domains, ensure a full justification for a partially non-sustainable option by the party proposing this option;
- avoid significant negative effects;
- ensure the future is protected (no transfer of negative effects to next generations) and;
- ensure explicit, open and sound arguments for the choices proposed (transparency).

Strong proposals that emerged from the case study included not introducing new vaccines into the weak EPI infrastructure, or doing so only after the infrastructure is improved. As the majority of stakeholders indicated, adding new vaccines in such an EPI infrastructure would mean, among other things, increased costs.

Step 8: Presenting the results and options to policy makers

This involves (OECD 2010):

- Presenting to policy- makers the results of SIA5 — and alternative policy options as mitigating measures in a transparent and understandable way.
- Providing both an overall view and an illustration of the major individual effects in the economic, environmental and social domains in the assessment presentation.
- Clarifying indirect impacts, presenting important conflicts, highlighting areas where mitigating measures are needed, indicating alternative approaches to mitigate the undesirable impacts, and presenting optimization opportunities.
- Presenting different options must include comparing and contrasting their (i) effectiveness — the extent to which the option can achieve the objectives of the proposal; (ii) efficiency — the extent to which the objectives can be achieved with a given level of resources; and (iii) consistency— the extent to which the option limits trade-offs across economic, environmental and social domains.
- Presenting assessment that includes an appropriate mixture of qualitative information and text along with graphics, tables and figures that can communicate a picture to decision-makers and other end-users quickly and effectively. They can clearly signal problematic impacts that require intervention.
- Illustrating assessment findings through approaches ranging from simple tables to more complicated multi-dimensional graphics and interactive software.

As Chapter 10 shows, the case study has used four dimensions for correct estimation of expenditure in the EPI: dimensions of sources, financing agents or intermediaries, providers, and functions, with corresponding NHAs tables (Tables 12, 13, 14 & 15) for presenting the results.

Implementing sustainable impact assessments (Practical Points):

This involves (OECD 2010):

- Executing SIA right at the beginning of the policy development. An SIA allows for better-informed decision making throughout the policy process and raises awareness of a wide range of policy challenges related to sustainable development.
- Symmetrizing and balancing by typically subjecting social, ecological and

economic impacts of policies to more detailed scrutiny than solely the one dimensional effects (e.g. ecological) of sectoral policies. SIA demands an integrated approach. In addition, a balanced input (formal or informal) by NGOs and experts from various sectors as well as business partners should be guaranteed.

- Enlarging framing by including the concerns of other departments or sectors and incorporating alternative, innovative and integrated policy options.
- Ensuring adequate quality assurance by safe-guarding sufficient "separation of powers" when installing the SIA process and procedures. For example, a conflict of interest can occur if the same people are responsible for deciding on the scope of the SIA, conducting the actual screening and then implementing the policy or plan.
- Ensuring sufficient capacity through sound and high quality assessment, especially of complex and far-reaching proposals which are demanding of time, resources and skills.
- Enhancing opportunities for learning. There is considerable potential for deliberation, social learning and innovation from a more open and pluralistic assessment process, which leads to better practice and more sound integrated policies, thereby enhancing sustainable development.

Many of these suggestions on implementing SIA are reflected in the case study example that Chapters 7-10 deal with. The study was conducted when the EPI was undergoing critical reforms and there was urgent need to inform the policy process. The study included approaches to obtain a wide-range of opinions from stakeholders. It provided opportunities to the researcher and his assistant for learning. However, there might have been some conflict of interest as the study was conducted entirely by the researcher and his assistant with the help of supervisors for mainly academic purposes, without all the required time, skills and resources.

Limitations/Challenges

There are several limitations or challenges for SIA that are outlined in the literature. As we have seen in chapter two (including box 12), one most important challenge for the concept of sustainability which, as indicated, is one of the three pillars of the SIA framework, concerns the different meanings ascribed to it specifically in healthcare within social development environments. This poses major methodological problems, such as the impossibility of empirically evaluating the outcomes of applying policies based on diverse conceptualizations of sustainability (Christopher et al, 2013). George et al

(2007) point to the problem of quantifying sustainability: many social, environmental and even economic aspects of sustainability are difficult to estimate quantitatively (and as we have seen, in some cases it may not even be desirable, for example, natural or social capital that may have an intrinsic value, that may not be quantifiable in monetary terms). Also SIA authors are faced with the challenge of lack of coherent, reliable and homogenous data (eg EC 2003). Box 32 outlines these and other important limitations/challenges for Sustainability Impact Assessment.

Box 32: Limitations/Challenges for Sustainability Impact Assessment
Generally, as Pope (2003) points out, integrated SIAs should be more than the sum of sectoral economic, social and environmental issues. This creates a number of questions regarding institutional and methodological issues. In terms of institutional issues, Dalal-Clayton & Sadler (2004) argue that this refers to the establishment of appropriate provisions and arrangements for SIAs within policy-making and planning processes. Therefore, SIAs should be made a "fundamental component of the decision-making process" (Pope, 2003, 8). Buselich (2002, summary) points out that, in practice, the most critical issue of SIA are "how environmental, social and economic information is analyzed, integrated and presented to decision-makers". Methodologically, SIAs also present new challenges. If SIAs are to integrate different policy issues into one assessment process, procedural and organizational provisions (which ministry is responsible, which other ministries and stakeholders will be included) as well as interdisciplinary approaches (acknowledging that single disciplinary approaches will not suffice) will need to be developed (Bond et al, 2001).

Source: Berger (2007)

Berger (2007) explain that it is because of such challenges that the European Commission already funded various research projects in order to gain insights into different methodologies for SIA (Tamborra, 2005, as cited by Berger 2007). An example is the MATISSE project, funded by the 6th Framework Programme for Research of the EU, whose aims are to enhance scientific knowledge on SIA and improve tools for integrated sustainability assessment (ISA). The objective is to support the development of cross-sectoral policies that deal with SD and explore ways policy regimes and institutional arrangements can be empowered (Weaver & Rotmans, 2006, as cited by Berger (2007).

Berger (2007) also states that to enhance international exchange, the OECD Horizontal Programme for SD in cooperation with the European Commission planned to hold a workshop on "sustainability assessment methodologies" in autumn 2007, in Amsterdam, Holland. The aims of the workshop were to identify best practices and develop guidelines for sustainability assessments. Participants would review the state-of-the-art in conducting integrated sustainability assessments and their policy application as a key tool for advancing SD.

Summary

This chapter has presented a description of the SIA framework, including its historical development, main features, process and steps, as well as some practical points on it implementation. The SIA framework allows for better-informed decision making throughout the policy process and raises awareness of a wide range of policy challenges related to sustainable development. Furthermore, it helps to reinforce existing debates and the quality and coherence of policy proposals; to set the agenda for sustainable development; to identify critical issues, such as future challenges and impacts; to show key trends and set priorities; to deliver results on the ground; to raise the level of dialogue and participation; and to increase transparency of the policy decision-making process at large. It can be applied to different targets, including policies, projects and regulations, and at different levels, including local, regional, national, and international. As a key decision-making tool, SIAs help to frame problems, identify policy impacts on all dimensions and scope solutions, In this sustainability impact assessments can contribute to the co-ordination and integration of policies and better governance for sustainable development. When implementing an SIA it important to start at the beginning of policy development; subject social, ecological and economic impacts of policies to more detailed scrutiny than solely the one dimensional effects; ensure adequate quality assurance; ensure sufficient capacity; and enhance opportunities for learning which, as we have seen, is crucial in dealing with the major limitations/challenges for SIA we outlined above. Despite its value as a policy tool, the SIA framework, like the stakeholder analysis and NHA frameworks, has limitations that must be considered by users of the approach. The next four chapters describe the case study example that included the principles of these methodological approaches, starting with the following chapter on the context in which the case study was applied.

7

Application Context

This chapter considers the context of the case study. The main aim of this chapter therefore is to demonstrate through the case study (Sarr 2005) the possibility of applying the SIA methodological approaches that include the Stakeholder Analysis Framework and Resource Map Strategy in immunization services. For this reason, the chapter firstly considers the profile of the Gambian context in which the study was developed and implemented. It then looks at the country's EPI including its management in which the methodological approaches were applied. The SIA methodology requires that an ex-ante analysis (which, as indicated, helps to give an idea of the future impact of a policy) should be based on a detailed, comprehensive and relevant description of the policy context, including detailed characterization of the major sectors involved (EU 2003).

Country Background

The Gambia, on the west coast of Africa, is one of the smallest countries on the African continent. It has a population of about 1.8 million (2013 census), growing at a rate of 2.7% per annum (GBoS 2017)and a Gross Domestic Product (GDP) of 2.1% in 2016 (ADB 2016). Ruled constitutionally, the country is divided into five administrative regions.

The government's current national development objectives and priorities accord high priority to the social sectors of health and education which give attention to child survival, protection and development programmes. The country has made some progress in achieving it health goals; though slow by comparison to its national vital indicators to other countries in the region.

The country's economy is predominantly agrarian with a low per-capita income of approximately US $330 per annum. Real GDP growth was estimated at 8 per-cent (MOF&ED 2005). The Human Development Index (HDI) was 0.452 with a ranking of 155 out of 177 countries (Hunan Development Report 2004). The 1998 poverty study indicated that 69% of the population is below the poverty line. The national debt stood at US$666 million in 2003 which is estimated to reach 764 million in 2004 (MOF&EA 2005). High inflation and exchange rate fluctuation have severely reduced household incomes particularly in the rural areas. The prices of food and other basic commodities, which are mostly imported, have also escalated with dramatic increases in the prices of staples and fuel.

In order to strengthen the involvement and participation of civil society, the government has embarked on the reform of the local government system in the form of decentralization. This will have an important impact on civil society and grassroots involvement in participatory planning and monitoring of programmes. In this regard, a divisional Sector –Wide Approach (SWAP) system, a method of working between government and donors, has been instituted. Within this approach is proposed a Divisional Development Fund which will serve as the repository of all funds derived from donors, the central government and locally generated revenue. Integrated divisional plans will be used as the basis for the allocation of the funds (FSP 2003).

The health system is organized around a three-tier system with increasing complexity in the type and range of services delivered. The Primary Health Care (PHC) or the Village Health Services (VHS) are community-based services co-financed by the government and the communities. The secondary/district level covers major health centres, minor health centres and dispensaries. Five main hospitals now constitute the tertiary level. The management of the health sector also follows a tree-tier system. To address the problem of a heavily centralized management system, the government embarked upon in 1993 reforms through structural changes in the Ministry that devolved administrative and management responsibilities to the Regional Health Teams (RHTs) to increase efficiency of service delivery at regional and community levels.

A new policy framework "Changing for Good" was produced to include new socio-economic and health development challenges to ensure access to essential quality health care to Gambians. Among the key issues identified are availability and access to essential drugs and vaccines, and partnership in the financing of health services.

The recurrent health expenditure, as a share of the total government expenditure, ranged from 10.8 to 13.4%, which represents real per-capita recurrent expenditure of US $ 3. 39 to US $ 5.91. In 2000, the recurrent expenditure on health as a proportion of GDP reached 11.17%, which was slightly below the average for sub-Saharan Africa. The public expenditure per-capita in the health sector in 2000 was US$ 6, which was just half of the recommended standard required to provide minimum health services (FSP 2003)

Both public and private providers provide health services. The private sector is expanding mainly with respect to out- patient care. Divisional health services are provided through:

- Major health centres
- Minor health centres
- Outreach clinics
- Community health posts
- Private providers in the region including traditional healers

In summary, this is the country background in terms of the impact of the country and health system context on the Gambian EPI programme. The following section looks at the Gambian EPI programme.

The Gambian EPI Programme

Delivery of immunization in an organised manner started in The Gambia as part of the West African Small Pox Eradication- Measles Programme. High rates of measles vaccination coverage in the 6-60-month-old target population were achieved through mobile teams operating from village to village. The transmission of measles was hindered for a period of two years. However, mobile operations were less effective in the identification and vaccination of new susceptible population groups and were stopped, mainly because of high costs. In 1979, The Gambia commenced the Expanded Programme on Immunization to provide BCG, DPT, poliomyelitis, measles, tetanus toxoid and yellow fever. Separate Expanded Programme on Immunization staff provided direction of EPI activities. The staff members were responsible for planning, training, logistics and evaluation. Because the mobile strategy was expensive and unsustainable, it was decided to use the Maternal and Child Health (MCH) teams to deliver immunization services to all the static and outreach immunization sites (Robertson et al, 1985).

In 2001 a coordinating committee, the Interagency Coordinating Committee (ICC), was instituted. This committee, which is chaired by the Director of Health Services, include officials of institutions outside the Department of State for Health & Social Welfare (DOSH&SW), such as MRC, the Gambia

Chamber of Commerce and Industry, UNICEF, WHO, Rotary International, EU and the African Development Bank (ADB). Since its inception, the ICC has taken up more responsibility for the total coordination for all the components of the programme, including National Immunization Days (NIDs) for Polio.

The ICC has these specific functions:

Coordinating all inputs and resources available from both inside and outside of the country, in order to maximize resources for the good of the child;

Assisting the EPI in resource mobilization and reviewing of the use of funds at regular intervals to enhance rational use, transparency and accountability;

Providing technical support and assisting in formulation of policy. The ICC supports the national level to review and endorse the work plans such as EPI five-year plans and surveillance plans;

Encouraging information sharing and feedback, not only at national level, but also at implementing levels within the country;

Advocating at national level for increased political commitment and for priority to be given to the EPI (EPI, DOSH&SW, 2001)

As a coordinating body the ICC has been considered by EPI staff to be effective in carrying out these functions. However, the ICC has been less effective in tackling the issue of instability of funding in the EPI and priority given to NIDs by donors because of several factors One factor which relates to its role is that the ICC, as an officer of a donor agency who sits on the ICC intimated, has not been very proactive in carrying out its advocacy and fundraising functions. According to this ICC member, a major weakness of the ICC is using donor funds without finding alternative sources of funding. The other factors are often beyond the control of the ICC. Availability of funding from donors, like UNICEF and WHO, are normally based on yearly funding plans that the DOSH&SW use to request foreign donors for funds. Such requests are sent through the donors' country office to the donors' headquarters abroad. At this level, donors like UNICEF mobilize funds through channels like the television and radio. Thus, ultimately the amount of funding that a country receives for its EPI from UNICEF, for example, would depend on the amounts UNICEF is able to mobilize. Also, there are special activities that donors give more emphasis and, therefore, more funding. Donors give priority to NIDs because such activities are aimed at meeting global health targets, which many donors like to be involved in.

Under the Vaccine Independent Initiative (VII), the Government in 1993 for the first time created a budget line for the procurement of vaccines and consumables amounting to US$ 131,275. At that time the health sector was reformed, leading to the creation of divisional health teams (DHTs) that were given the responsibility of managing the decentralized health services. However, the decentralization process had little impact on immunization services, as the DHTs lack autonomy with regard to the deployment of staff and financial matters.

Since its inception, the EPI programme has been able to steadily increase immunization coverage within the target population to the coverage rate of 80% of fully immunized children less than one year old. To maintain this coverage level and to further increase coverage and the immunization services in 1995 the DOSH&SW decided to involve the private clinics in the provision of immunization services (Gambia EPI Review, 2001).

While the general objective of the EPI is to reduce childhood morbidity and mortality due to EPI targeted diseases (tuberculosis, hepatitis B, poliomyelitis, diphtheria, pertussis, tetanus, haemophilus Influenzae type B, measles and yellow fever), the programme aims to realize the following general objectives in the five years following the implementation of the Financial Sustainability Plan (FSP) that was prepared in 2003:

- To raise the awareness among Gambians on the benefits of immunization and the consequences of failing to get children vaccinated at the right time
- To maintain high immunization coverage
- To ensure the sustainable availability and delivery of vaccines in the programme
- To strengthen and improve the disease surveillance system with special emphasis on the EPI targeted diseases
- To ensure injection safety in the EPI delivery system

Specifically the objectives are:

- To increase immunization coverage to 95% and above for all the antigens
- To increase to 90% fully immunized children under one year
- To prevent stock-outs of all EPI antigens at all levels and improve the effectiveness of the purchasing system
- To reduce measles morbidity and mortality by 90% and 95% respectively
- To maintain the elimination level of neonatal tetanus to less than 1 case per 1,000 live births in every division
- To eradicate poliomyelitis by the year 2008
- To reduce vaccine wastage to the target levels specified in the costing in Section 4
- To immediately strengthen the cold chain by increasing capital investment for the replacement of old equipment and by adopting a policy of solarization.

- To integrate in a sustainable manner the Pneumococcal vaccine, if the current trial proves successful, into the routine EPI in 2007
- To develop posters on EPI targeted diseases and the vaccination schedule
- To develop key messages on immunization targeting parents and caregivers
- To continue to use auto-disposable (AD) syringes for all EPI vaccinations
- To ensure the use and proper disposal of safety boxes by all facilities conducting immunization services
- Cutts et al (2005) conducted during the period 2002-2004 a randomized, placebo-controlled, double-blind trial in eastern Gambia to assess the efficacy of a nine-valent (having a valency or strength of nine) pneumococcal conjugate vaccine in children. The results demonstrate that pneumococcal conjugate vaccine has high efficacy against radiological (relating to the science of X-rays and other high-energy radiation) pneumonia and greatly decreases admissions and improves child survival.

This is the second study assessing the efficacy of a pneumococcal conjugate vaccine in The Gambia. During the period 2001-2004 the MRC in collaboration with The Gambia government conducted a trial for a seven-valent pneumococcal conjugate vaccine that is more efficacious than the nine-valent vaccine (the nine valent is two-valents less efficacious than the seven-valent) in preventing radiological pneumonia in the Gambia. However, the seven-valent vaccine will not be introduced in the Gambia in the near future because it has limited market. Instead, the less efficacious nine-valent vaccine is planned to be introduced in the Gambia because it has a very large market in South Africa and the USA where trials have also found the vaccine to be efficacious against invasive pneumococcal disease.

The Gambian EPI has been shown to be highly cost-effective (e.g. WDR, 1993; Hinman, 1999; Brenzel, 1989; Robertson, 1985). Using the estimated immunization effects in terms of cases and deaths prevented and the immunization costs of the programme, Robertson et al (1985) calculated two cost-effective indicators, namely, cost per case prevented and cost per death prevented. The cost-effectiveness analyses show a range of cost per case prevented by immunization from $1.30 for pertussis and $1.96 for measles to over $650 for poliomyelitis and $890 for diphtheria. The cost per death prevented ranges from about $40 for measles to $6,555 for poliomyelitis and $11,133 for diphtheria.

The findings of an intensive study (Hall et al, 1992) of the costs and cost-effectiveness of the EPI show that the total and average costs of the full national EPI fell impressively from about US$1.5 per dose in the early 1980s to

$0.6 in 1988, and a large decline in cost per fully immunized child from about US$ 19.0 to US$5.6. When compared with earlier findings of the programme, and with figures from other developing countries, the Gambian EPI appears highly cost-effective for 1988 (Hall et al, 1992). More recently estimation of the costs of the EPI in 1998 (Kodjo et al, 2001) indicates that the total cost of EPI implementation was around US$ 720, 551 and the average cost of US$ 0.6 per dose and US$37 per fully immunized child (FIC).

The country successfully introduced two new vaccines over a period of ten years: Hepatitis B and DPT- Hib (Haemophilus influenzae type b is a type of bacteria that can cause a number of different illnesses, ranging from skin infections to more serious problems like blood infections or meningitis). In order to introduce the two new vaccines the Government implemented changes including estimation of additional cold chain space required for the new vaccines and procurement of appropriate cold chain equipment; training of staff on the new schedule and sensitization and awareness creation for the media and caregivers on the new vaccines (Gambia EPI Review, 2001)

Prior to the introduction of the new vaccines disease burden studies were successfully conducted to establish the need for the new vaccines. The Medical Research Council, UK, in collaboration with the Gambia government and the International Agency for Research on Cancer had instituted The Gambia Hepatitis Intervention Study with the aim of assessing whether prevention of chronic liver cancer, particularly hepatocellular carcinoma would be achieved through the prevention of persistent infection with Hepatitis B virus by immunization. The study consisted of three phases: (1) integration of Hepatitis immunization into the Expanded Programme on Immunization (2) evaluation of the immunogenicity of the vaccine and the duration of protection. This needs the long- term follow-up of a cohort of 1000 immunized children and (3), determination of the incidence of chronic liver disease in the vaccinated and the unvaccinated (Hall, 1990).

However, there were several challenges that were associated with the introduction of the new vaccines, such as lack of a long-term vaccine financing plan for routine and new vaccines, lack of a plan on the replacement of aging cold chain equipment, and frequent breakdown of transport used for outreach services (Gambia EPI Review 2001).

Summary

This chapter has looked at the context in which the case study methodology was applied, including The Gambia's EPI. The EPI, both internationally and in The Gambia, has proved to be one of the most successful public health interventions in the past 20 years, as shown by the cost-effectiveness of the vaccines. But the pressure to expand the EPI by adding to its new vaccines, which is a result of the success the programme has registered over the years, has serious implications for the sustainability of the EPI. This is a policy challenge that led to the development of the case study methodological approach which we now consider in the following chapter.

8

The Case Study Methodological Approach

As indicated in Chapter 6, step 3 of the SIA framework, Selecting Tools or Methodologies, the necessity of combining tools is important for integrated assessment, and a precondition for devising efficient tool combinations is to know the tools which exist and the analytical results they can provide. As mentioned, the study (Sarr, 2005) on which the methodological approach is based assesses the sustainability of the expansion of the Expanded Programme on Immunization (EPI) in The Gambia, and explores whether to use additional resources for improving efficiency in the supply chain or introduce new vaccines which, as mentioned, has been the government policy. As indicated, the objectives of the study were to identify appropriate tools for measuring the sustainability of the provision of immunization services, institutional and behavioural factors which affect the efficiency and sustainability of the immunization service and policy recommendations for improving or maintaining the level of immunization services. Here the term "methodology" (or methodological) refers to the systematic, theoretical analysis of the methods applied to assessing the sustainability of immunization programmes. It includes concepts like paradigm, theoretical model, phases and quantitative and qualitative techniques (Irny et al 2005). The methodological approach used here provides theoretical foundation for understanding which method, set of methods or best practices can be applied to assessing the sustainability of immunization programmes in especially the contexts of developing countries. It allows for the systematic study of methods that are, can be, or have been applied within a discipline, the study or description of methods, and the analysis of the principles of methods, rules, and postulates used by the discipline.

A literature review demonstrates that there were no existing, appropriate tools for the objectives and, therefore, new tools were developed: a stakeholder analysis questionnaire and a resource map tool. The Stakeholder Analysis Framework and the Resource Map Strategy which mainly constitute the methodological approach are useful processes for policy related research but their use in immunization contexts to assess the sustainability of the introduction of new vaccines is lacking. The chapter starts with the rationale of the methodological approach. Then, it outlines the goal, objectives, questions and conceptual framework of the study on which the methodological approach is based. Finally, the chapter outlines in more detail the structure of the methodological approach.

Rationale

The Expanded Programme on Immunization (EPI) was established in 1974 to develop and expand immunization programmes throughout the world. The term was used because until then, most immunization programmes had only used smallpox, BCG and diphtheria, tetanus and pertussis (DPT) vaccines. New vaccines were included in the EPI, covering six diseases. These are diphtheria, neonatal tetanus, poliomyelitis, measles, tuberculosis and whooping cough. The basis for the selection was the high burden of disease and the availability of a well-tried vaccine for which the price is available. By the early 1990s most countries began health sector reforms during which the achievements and setbacks became clear (World Bank 1993). In developing countries the objective of the reforms focused on enhancing the efficiency and financing of health systems (WHO 2000). Decentralization and integration of vertical programmes such as EPI were the concentrations of the reforms in many of these countries. The intentions of the EPI reforms in dealing with financing, decentralization, and integration of some generic functions have generally been seen as admirable.

However, because of the success of the EPI, there has been an obvious pressure to utilize the infrastructure more, by adding new vaccines to the EPI. Potentially highly efficacious new vaccines against diarrheal and respiratory diseases could have an impact on the burden of these diseases, which has been estimated to be as high as 8 million deaths per annum worldwide (Batson, 1998).

These vaccines that are also important in terms of public-health perspectives are particularly geared toward children of developing countries where the burden of disease is high. Particularly in these countries, childhood immunization is seen as a key channel for the achieving the Millennium Development Goal 4 (MDG 4) of reducing child mortality by two-thirds within 2015.

However, most developing countries lack the resources to access, evaluate, and implement these newly-developed vaccines. For example, despite the widespread nature of the disease, immunization for Hepatitis B is not always readily available in many developing countries like The Gambia, due to financial constraints (Hall et al, 1993), poor public and medical knowledge, lack of information on vaccine efficacy, insufficient health infrastructure and the changing priorities of international donors (USGAO, 1999). Information obtained from several other countries (often point to problems such as unanticipated costs, incomplete planned assessments and preparatory actions, insufficient time, and a lack of appreciation of the complexity of good preparations. Most interestingly, it was found that although country wealth and the strength of the pre-introduction EPI components were no doubt important, there were several instances when even middle-income countries with strong EPIs encountered high stress from new and underutilized vaccines (NUVIs).

Also more recent evidence from many countries (eg Shearer 2012) suggests a great need for increased cold chain capacity. The importance of training and education for health care workers and social mobilization is frequently indicated. Also suggested are the needs for tapping potential for wider partnerships and strategies within the Ministry of Health (MOH). It appeared that important determinants of smooth or disruptive introductions were the choice of a vaccine, presentation, formulation, and packaging as well as the quality and thoroughness of pre-introduction planning and actions.

Many developing countries like The Gambia in particular depend to a large extent on donor funding from sources such as UNICEF and GAVI (Global Alliance for Vaccines and Immunization) for their programme and this can result in inconsistent level of funding from one year to the next, depending on the donor priorities and programming. The literature (eg Favin et al 2012) shows several consequences of this situation: failure by some countries to plan for collateral costs like endured expansion of cold and dry storage capacity; fuel for running the cold chain (often in local budgets); and a frequent and higher-volume distribution of vaccines and related supplies. In addition to these problems, countries that had almost reached the end date of donor financing had no solution for how new vaccine costs would continue to be paid. Although there is much international attention, as well as some positive moves such as co-financing and reduced Pneumococcal conjugate vaccine (PCV) prices for GAVI-eligible countries, they could not afford the cost of new vaccines (plus their distribution and storage) without donor support. Countries that are eligible for GAVI support do not enjoy some price-reduction mechanisms, making them as a result encounter much financial constraints to introducing new vaccines. These countries were required to increase their vaccine allocations by a factor of 6.8 from 2004-8. Thus, long-term financing of new vaccines and their impact on the limited national health budgets are crucial issues.

In addition to the problem of ensuring funding for immunization with current vaccines, countries must make decisions on whether it can afford new vaccines or whether it should mobilize any such funds to increase coverage. The literature (eg Favin et al 2012) also shows that the likelihood that NUVI will strengthen EPI and health system components appears to be related to specific planning for these outcomes and to taking a long-term view to system strengthening, a critical requirement that is often lacking in the examples from the many countries studied.

The new vaccines differ from those originally included in the Expanded Programme on Immunization (EPI) in at least two ways: they tend to be largely more expensive than current vaccines, together with the fact that some targeted diseases are relatively underestimated and, thus, the demand for them by the political view and public may be absent. The slow introduction and uptake of new vaccines makes it more important for providing policymakers the required information for making decisions.

After the new vaccines are licensed, policymakers require information on, among other things, the burden of disease, costs of vaccines, and cold-chain facilities to make decision to introduce new vaccines. But the decision-making process can be complex, particularly because it involves many actors and is pushed by multiple factors. Increasing the understanding of the decision-making process in the introduction of new vaccines helps establish why vaccines are adopted or not and contributes to building a sustainable demand for vaccines in a country (Akumu et al 2007).

On what influences decisions on the introduction of new vaccines, there is evidence from many developing countries (e.g., Akumu et al 2007) to show that the burden of disease, findings of research on vaccine-preventable diseases, political issues relating to outbreaks of certain diseases, initiatives of international and local stakeholders, pressure from the development partners, GAVI's support, and financial matters are main considerations in the introduction of new vaccines in many countries. Perhaps the most important factor in developing countries in speeding up the introduction and uptake of new vaccines is GAVI's quick approval of applications from countries for its support, as well as the countries taking less time to meet the administrative requirements.

The addition of new vaccines to the EPI is an agreeable policy but should only be considered where the infrastructure is capable of sustaining both it and any additional vaccines, and where it is the best use of limited immunization resources. In some circumstances, countries may be better off using their limited resources to strengthen or improve the EPI in order to reach more children. The term is used in various ways; however a good policy usually has these main characteristics: it includes topics of principles; it concentrates on action, indicating what needs to be done and who is to do it; it is a prescriptive statement made by a group or an individual with the prerogative to do so. Most importantly, a good policy serves as a tool that permits people to conduct the main functions of an organization more effectively and efficiently and makes its administration lighter.

To help policymakers make such critical decisions future evaluations of new vaccine introductions should include the systematic and objective assessment of the impacts on a country's immunization system and broader health system, especially in lower-income countries. There are at least three benefits of such health impact assessment (which, as indicated, includes Sustainability Impact Assessment) : Improving the evidence.- explicitly identifying data gaps and evidence needed to improve future assessments, stimulating policy-relevant scientific research more directly, whether to develop new empirical studies or to improve systematic evaluation and synthesis of existing evidence, and providing valuable new data directly relevant to answering policy-relevant causal questions that often cannot be addressed with observational studies or randomized trials; Raising awareness among policy-makers and the public-contributing to a more comprehensive understanding of the causes of illness and of the role of policies, programs, projects, and plans in shaping health outcomes, including strategies that are likely to make the most difference in improving health and in reducing health disparities. A new paradigm for productive collaborations-providing opportunities for a new paradigm for productive collaborations by offering opportunities (1) for scientists to be more directly involved in the application of the science that they conduct to improve public health and to be made more aware of the type of evidence needed for policy decisions, (2) for identification of new data sources and designs needed to answer important scientific and policy-relevant questions, (3) for improved ability of policy-makers to consider health implications in making decisions and improved understanding of the links between policies and health, (4) for active participation of community members in decision-making and increased access to information on health consequences available through the assessment process, which can enhance their ability to advocate for health, and (5) for improved insights into the potential pathways through which proposed decisions are likely to affect the health of residents (National Academy of Sciences 2011).

There is a clear need for a framework to ensure a standardized and consistently applied methodology for decision making. The use of such a framework would minimize excess mortality, maximize resources, reduce wastage, ensure equity, and ultimately improve accountability to the population at risk and other stakeholders. This demand requires a process that involves key agencies to ensure a pragmatic and feasible approach to development of tools that provide the needed information to EPI policy processes.

However, assessing the sustainability of policies, programmes, projects, and plans is a challenge that requires not only the collaboration of scientists, policy -makers, and communities, but also an interdisciplinary approach that involves such disciplines as health, social sciences, economics, and policy. Systematic processes for rigorously assessing health consequences are needed. Although numerous analytic and deliberative tools are being used to incorporate aspects of health into decisions, none fully provides all the necessary attributes (National Academy of Sciences 2011).

The case study methodological approach (Sarr, 2005) for assessing the sustainability of immunization programmes can help policy-makers in diverse contexts, particularly developing countries; make decisions on the sustainability issue of whether to use additional resources for improving efficiency in the supply chain rather than introducing new vaccines, which has been the policy of many governments. It can contribute to the process of identifying a better understanding of the long-term sustainability of the EPI with regard to this issue. Using this approach will help to identify where sustainability issues may arise if external funding agencies withdraw their support or if the MOH budget resources are cut. In addition it will assist in identifying the sources of funding for the programme and the mix of current financing strategies and their success in mobilizing sufficient resources in the country (Levine et al, 2001). Also the approach helps to describe in detail the flow of resources and expenditures and how they are used within a health system. When assessing health care strategies and policies, there is generally a lack of information on the management and the political process involved. The approach also uses the strategy of resource mapping to organize and compile data that focus on questions of power, relationships, processes and accountability in the EPI.

While the good intentions of the EPI reforms in dealing with financing, decentralization, and integration of some generic functions are admirable, the reform process itself may be questionable. Sometimes the reform process can trigger opposition from the stakeholders, a situation that could constrain the force of implementation of a good programme in many ways, including decrease in previous achievements and reversion of reforms. Thus, the situation analyses that come before the reform should identify the interests of each of the stakeholders with the aim of making proper changes in the reform process. This is consistent with the suggestion (Walt 1994) that policy-makers should be involved in research processes if the result of research are to feed into policy or are to be used by policy-makers. This methodological approach uses a process of systematically gathering and analyzing qualitative information from stakeholders to determine whose interests should be taken into account when developing, reforming and/or implementing a policy or programme, but more importantly the process assesses where people think the system works and where it doesn't work, and if different parties have contradictory incentives.

The standard techniques of stakeholder analysis and national health accounting are adapted to the methodological approach. The approach also incorporates in the stakeholder analysis framework selected indicators of financial sustainability from the literature (GAVI 2000), together with country-specific indicators in the Stakeholder Analysis framework. Using these tools one can obtain data from the EPI, government and donor records, and conduct interviews with stakeholders at the central, divisional and facility levels.

This methodological approach to assessing immunization programmes is derived from a 3-year study (Sarr 2005) at London South Bank University, UK, that focused on assessing the sustainability of the expansion of the Expanded Programme on Immunisation EPI in The Gambia, and explores whether to use additional resources for improving efficiency in the supply chain rather than introducing new vaccines, which has been the government policy. The objectives of the study were to identify appropriate tools for measuring the financial sustainability of the provision of immunization services, institutional and behavioural factors which affect the efficiency and sustainability of the immunization service and policy recommendations for improving or maintaining the level of immunization services.

The sustainability of complex EPI programmes depends on many technical and organizational issues that need to be properly addressed by a sustainability policy. For purpose of our discussion, we define a sustainability policy as a document that states what is and what is not allowed in an immunization system to advance its sustainability. It consists of a set of rules that could be expressed in formal, semi-formal or very informal language. In many contexts, an immunization system can be considered sustainable and efficient if the policy enforced by its administrators is well-informed and trustworthy too; from this standpoint it is possible to evaluate the system sustainability by evaluating its policy.

The methodological approach aims to provide a framework for formalizing and comparing policies, and a sustainability approach to evaluate the sustainability level of immunization systems that are expanding through the introduction of new vaccines. All the components of the methodological approach are illustrated by applying it to a real case study from the Gambian EPI. The Gambia is well known for having achieved very high immunization coverage at a low cost. Nonetheless, many changes in coverage and funding levels were identified in succeeding years, suggesting that there is a potential for improving efficiency and sustainability. In addition, a future GAVI and other international donor policies play an inordinately large part in the future of the Gambian EPI, and as such the system of financing must remain flexible. The study therefore focused on the following guiding aim, objectives, questions and conceptual framework.

Aim, objectives and questions of the study

Aim

To assess the sustainability of the expansion of the Expanded Programme on Immunization in The Gambia.

Specific objectives

- To identify appropriate tools for measuring the financial sustainability (as broadly defined in Chapter Two) of the provision of immunization services in The Gambia;
- To identify institutional and behavioural factors which affect the efficiency and sustainability of immunization services;
- To identify policy recommendations for improving or maintaining the level of immunization services in The Gambia.

Questions

The questions of the study are:

1. Is the Expanded Programme on Immunization (EPI) sustainable?
2. Is the funding sustainable?
3. How does adding vaccines affect sustainability?

Conceptual framework of the study

Definitions of health care financing and sustainability

Health care financing generally refers to the resources used to provide health care. This includes money as well as other resources such as gifts in kind. Its main affairs are how money is raised, who controls it, and how it is spent. However, the impact of these questions goes beyond money matters. The ways by which a health service is financed will have far-reaching implications for the way it is delivered and the care it gives. Therefore, health care financing is an essential issue in health services delivery.

A closely related concept is that of Sector-Wide Approaches (SWAPs) (Cassels 1997) to health financing. Sector-Wide Approaches are methods of working between government and donors. All significant funding for the sector support a single sector policy and expenditure programme under government leadership, adopting common approaches across the sector and relying on government procedures to disburse and account for all funds. In contrast, traditional donor-driven project based funding approaches often absorb scarce human and financial resources in activities with limited coverage, adopting standards that cannot be replicated or sustained and relying heavily on expatriate technical assistance that is unhelpful to the development of local capacity. At the heart of the SWAPs approach is a medium-term programme of work dealing with the development of sectoral policies and strategies; projections of resource availability and plans of expenditures. Additionally, it is necessary to establish processes and structures for negotiating strategic and management questions, and reviewing sectoral performance against targets and milestones that both donors and governments agree upon.

As we have seen, there are several definitions of sustainability, each emphasizing various authority on the sustainability of health care. The definitions generally refer to the capacity of a system to survive with a specific level of external support. The concept does not necessarily mean self-sufficiency, or depending entirely on one's own strength and resources. However, it does mean self-reliance which outlines a community's initiative in taking responsibility for their own health development. Self-reliance is unlike self-sufficiency. Whereas self-sufficiency emphasizes entire dependence on a country's own capabilities and resources, self-reliance stresses a country's ability to mobilize and allocate sufficient domestic and external resources on a reliable basis to realize immunization performance targets.

Also, we have seen that although a particular emphasis is put on the economic aspect of sustainability, where financing matters play a major part, several other factors influence the long-term sustainability of a health programme than merely its financial security and stability. These include the managerial and technical capacity of the programme and the external environment in which it functions, staff motivation, currency valuation, and the economic and political climate surrounding the programme, both locally and internationally (Goodman et al 1993)

Financial sustainability has been often applied to situations where external funders tried to encourage governments of developing countries to mobilize domestic resources for health programmes that had been funded previously by donors. However, more than for many other health programmes, the characteristics of immunization and the interest shown by international bodies in the future success of immunization programmes may demand that the focus of financial sustainability be shifted toward the ability of a country to mobilize and allocate sufficient domestic and external resources on a reliable basis to achieve target levels of immunization programmes. The emphasis therefore moves from the attention to phasing out external funding, and toward the issue of how to structure the total package of financing and use available resources efficiently to ensure that sufficient funds are available on a reliable basis (Levine, et al 2001)

Sustainability of the EPI and current international initiatives

We have seen in Chapter 2 that some have viewed self-sufficiency as the ultimate goal of achieving sustainable financing. However, in the nearer term sustainable financing is seen by others as the ability of a country to mobilize and efficiently use domestic and supplementary external resources on a reliable basis to achieve target levels of immunization performance. Such immunization performance includes current and future goals for access, utilization, quality, safety and equity (WHO, 2001).

Thus, the debate on financial sustainability of the EPI has often focused on extended discussion on sources of funds. In developing countries, the financing challenge has traditionally been met, in part, by external aid: grant funds for vaccine procurement, health service infrastructure, training of health personnel, and other inputs. However, external support for immunization programmes has proven to be no more reliable than domestic sources of financing because of the ever- changing volume and orientation of donor support.

The sources of funds may influence the profile of what type and quality of service are available, and where, and by whom they are used and thus the sustainability of the EPI. For example, whereas cost sharing together with social mobilisation is seen by many as an effective way of generating funds for health programmes, such as immunization, it is argued (Kremer et al 2003) that cost sharing is inappropriate when there are large externalities (economists define externalities as positive or negative effects of an activity that do not appear as direct costs or benefits to the individual or organization undertaking the activity and thus do not influence project decision-making). The term "impact" is often used interchangeably with the term "externality"). What may be required to sustain such services including their use, it is further argued, are large external subsidies.

It is argued that grant-making and lending institutions are likely to be contributing to the financing of immunization services over the foreseeable future, and can provide that support in ways that are likely to foster long-term sustainability. However, it is argued that unless funding for immunization is buffered from both domestic and international political processes it will not be possible to attain true financial sustainability (Levine et al, 2001).

As we have seen, the debate about sustainability has, therefore, often called attention to how long-term trends affect a transition to sustainability. The nature of trends which each includes a trend that makes a sustainable transition more feasible as well as trends that make it more difficult has been explored (Kates et al 2003). The classes of trends are: (1) peace and security, (2) population, migration and urbanization, (3) affluence, poverty, well-being and health (4) production, consumption and technology, (5) globalization, governance, and institutions, and (6) global environmental change (land, oceans, atmosphere, rapid environmental change and changing problems) (Kates et al 2003). According to Kates et al (2003) some long-term trends in nature and society serve as currents along which we can navigate directions towards a 21st century sustainability transition. This transition is seen by Kates et al (2003) as one where a stabilizing world population meets its needs, reduces hunger and poverty, while maintaining the planet's life support systems and living resources. Hastening favourable trends, slowing harmful trends, understanding complex trends, and noting changes in direction and form that compose significant departures is considered by Kates et al as a great challenge of sustainability science. In many developing countries, if the mix of favourable and unfavourable trends continue at the current pace, it is unlikely that a future transition will be realized. The current pace of meeting such human needs as feeding, housing and employing the growing populations while improving, is well beyond the pace needed to realize targets in areas like immunization. Hence the need for continued donor support to sustain immunization programmes.

The long-term trends might influence the transition to sustainability of the EPI in several ways. Wars, conflicts, crime and corruption pose major threats to sustainability of the EPI by directly destroying human lives, capital, infrastructure and environment, and indirectly by, among things, diverting needed productive resources for the EPI. Population numbers, location and trends influence the sustainability of the EPI in terms of the numbers of humans whose immunization needs are to be met and the driving force of threats to the EPI through its resource use. Meeting human needs for immunization of a much larger population requires growth in affluence and economy (income and wealth) and its distribution in ways that reduce hunger and poverty. Also, favourable shifts in factors like investment and income in interconnected developed or donor countries may be accompanied by, among other things, unpredictable withdrawal of capital, adding new sources of instability in the EPI of poor countries.

The discussion on sustainability of the EPI has also concentrated on the use of funds for immunization. For instance, because of the cost of National Immunization Days (NIDs) and because they have to be implemented intensively, NIDs tend to be, among other things, donor driven and coercive. There has been a controversy over NIDs that they are diverse; they limit resources and hamper the existing other immunizations. On the other hand, some writers (eg Adachi et al 1999 and Melgaard et al 2005) suggest that the positive effects are limited only when the campaigns are frequently repeated or only where the infrastructure has been installed. Although goal-oriented NIDs can motivate health workers, the motivation for routine immunization may be hampered. These negative effects may result in the low intention to sustain vaccination activities. There is some documented evidence of vaccination failures after NIDs (Adachi et al 1999).

Capital costs represent a small portion of all expenditures needed to maintain immunization systems, but are required for cold chain or other necessary infrastructure. However, it is argued that restricting external funding to capital investments does not contribute to reaching the objectives of financial sustainability (Levine et al 2001). Donors must direct their resources to meeting the costs of recurrent items like allowances of health workers, not only to capital investments which they typically prefer to do (e.g. Kremer et al 2003, Simms et al 200).

A related and equally strong concern comes from those who see the need for serious consideration of the human resource and other non-financial requirements of the EPI (eg Simms et al 2005, Melgaard et al 1999). For instance, Melgaard et al argue that even in countries where the planning of human resources produces the proper number and mix of personnel, the effectiveness of eradication programmes like immunization is often affected by the low performance that characterize the under-funded public sector. This lowers the productivity of the health workers. There is therefore stress on the need for immunization programmes to utilize and work within the frame of the existing health system to increase the support to national health development in critical areas like human resources development, capacity building, infrastructure development, and service management and delivery so as to increase the impact on the health status of the population.

The debate over using funds for the introduction of new vaccines in the EPI is one of the most controversial of recent times. Such debate has often focused on the narrow discussion of the cost-effectiveness of new vaccines and the need for their use as rapidly as possible (eg Widdus 1999). Many health professionals and the public think that there are important factors to consider other than the cost-effectiveness of new vaccines (Widdus 1999). For instance, it is argued (e.g. Dasgupta et al 1999) that in situations of decreasing social sector spending in a resource constrained economy currently undergoing structural adjustment resources will not be easy to come by. Considering the low health budgets of many developing countries, how justified will such additional expenditure is on just one disease (e.g. Hepatitis B) with epidemiological priority. Experience so far suggests that choosing to introduce new vaccines can significantly increase the cost of the EPI (eg Kadder et al 2004; Sarr 2005). Furthermore, other interventions that limit transmission in the social and professional processes may require much less financial input, but much more human interaction to change attitudes and lead to more "sustainable" results (e.g. Dasgupta et al 1999).

In many respects, the issue of introducing new vaccines in developing countries provides a window through which many have examined a range of public -private partnership issues on sustainability of the EPI. Here the controversy is fundamentally about the pros and cons of such public-private partnerships (e.g. Mills et al 2005). While the discussion often concentrates on the role and activities of private providers of services, perhaps the main focus is on the Global Alliance for Vaccines and Immunization (GAVI). GAVI aims to introduce new and underused vaccines and increase EPI coverage in 74 developing countries globally. It provides safe injection equipment, new vaccines and small financial support for an initial five-year funding period. By the end of 2001, 52 countries had been approved for $134 million of funding (Brugha et al 2002). While it is argued that the challenge of financing the EPI has recently been brought into high relief by the availability of funding under GAVI and the funding demands associated with new vaccine technologies (Levine et al 2001), many criticisms have been leveled against GAVI (e.g. Hardon 2005, Edmunds et al 2005, Brugha et al 2002). For example, on the issue of equity within countries, it is argued that countries will not be able to achieve one of the objectives of GAVI, which is that 80% of countries should reach 80% coverage in all districts, if the organization continues to spend around two-thirds of its resources on procurement and supply of new vaccines, rather than strengthening of immunization services. That, as Simms et al (2002) suggests, "efforts to tackle major diseases will be unsustainable in the long term unless action is first taken to establish effective health systems". It is further argued that "sector-wide approaches" that encourage governments to decentralize and reform health planning and management and which have tremendous potential to contribute to sustainability are a better way of strengthening health systems than separate donor-driven vertical programmes, such as those supported by GAVI. Such approaches meet the need to set targets for financial sustainability in a participatory fashion with full inputs from experts and policy-makers in recipient countries.

The criticisms against GAVI seem to focus particularly on the consequences of its Global Fund for sustainability. For example, it is argued (Waddington 2004) that it should not be assumed that earmarked donor funding, such as the Global Fund, automatically increases the allocation of developing-country resources towards programmes with the greatest health benefits. The allocation of such resources is not always increased because this is influenced by how the funding is designed. This is true especially in the longer term, once the earmarked funds have ended. Even in the short term, total funding does not necessary increase due to fungibility (ie governments that receive funding adjust their spending to offset donor funding preferences). Such problems that are associated with earmarked funds have been explored (Waddington 2004): earmarking does not agree with the spirit of the sector-wide approach; earmarking can lead governments to accept interventions which they cannot afford in the longer term; local ownership of an activity is often compromised; from the national perspective, it makes sense not to double-fund activities; the situation for decision makers is confused by the many earmarked funds.

Health policy

Most people see health policy as that which is concerned with content, which, for example, is about the preferred method of financing health services, or about improving a kind of health care. However, health policy is also about process and power. It is interested in who influences whom in the formulation of policy, and how that happens. It involves political systems, power and influence and the participation of people in policy making

The preferred way to understand health policy is to look at both processes and power - exploring the role of the state, both nationally and internationally, the actors in the state, the external forces pressuring it, and the mechanisms in the political system for participation in policy formulation. This extracts from societal-centred approaches as well as state- centred approaches, putting them in a global context (Walt, 1994).

Framework for the sustainability of the EPI

The above discussion demonstrates that the issue of sustainability of the EPI cannot be divorced from the social (including political), economic and environmental climate surrounding a health programme, both in the local context, and in the wider national and international context. As Figure 6 shows, threats to the sustainability of the EPI, for example, are government bureaucratic procedures, poor economic conditions in a country, currency devaluation, unfavourable political climate and long-term global trends.

The development of the methodological approach that the next chapter deals with was guided by this conception of how all these social, economic and environmental factors influence the sustainability of the EPI.

Development of the Methodological Approach

As already mentioned, the methodological approach was developed to address several issues of sustainability in the EPI sufficiently, and answer the questions of the case study on which it is based. It consists mainly of a Stakeholder Analysis Framework (Schmeer 1999) that has been identified from the literature for adoption, and a Resource Map strategy. As already mentioned, the stakeholder analysis uses a process of systematically gathering and analysing qualitative information from stakeholders (actors- persons or organisations - who have a vested interest in a policy or programme that is being promoted) to determine whose interests should be taken into account when developing and/or implementing a policy or programme. Selected indicators of financial sustainability in two immunisation assessment tools, namely, the Financial Immunisation tool (Levine et al 2001) and the WHO Common Assessment tool (WHO 2002), together with country-specific indicators, are incorporated in the Stakeholder Analysis questionnaire. The Resource Map questionnaire has been developed and used with stakeholders to complement the Stakeholder Analysis tool. The resource map strategy describes in detail the flow of resources and expenditures and how they are used within a system on the basis of the National Health Accounts methodology outlined in detail in chapter 5. As indicated, National Health Accounts (NHA) is an internationally standardised methodology for measuring financial resource flows in the health sector. It is a tool that allows countries to track the flow of health spending from financial sources to end users, and can be used to capture general health and disease-specific expenditures. The results of NHA studies can dictate the development of a health financing policy

The methodological approach focuses on the analysis of stakeholder characteristics and definitions (Schmeer 1999): interests in the issue of whether to use additional resources for improving the EPI infrastructure and funding and not for introducing new vaccines will help policy-makers and managers better understand the stakeholder's position and possible ways of addressing his/her concerns. It is crucial to identify possible stakeholder alliances because alliances can make a weak stakeholder stronger, or provide an avenue to influence several stakeholders by dealing with a single stakeholder. For the same reason, it is also important to determine the stability of stakeholder alliances. The amount of resources that a stakeholder has and his/her ability to mobilise such resources and the durability of such stakeholder power are an important characteristic that will determine the force with which the stakeholder might support or oppose the issue of whether to use additional resources for improving the EPI infrastructure, not for introducing new vaccines. Knowing whether or not a stakeholder has leadership will assist policy-makers and managers focus on those stakeholders who will be more inclined to actually show their support for or against the issue of whether to use additional resources for improving the EPI infrastructure and not for introducing new vaccines and convince others to do so. Added to these adopted generic characteristics is the stakeholder's agreement or disagreement on the indicators of sustainability, and his/her opinion on the extent to which the actions have been taken or implemented by Government. Knowing what indicators stakeholders consider important and the extent to which the actions have been implemented will help the country propose in its financial sustainability plans country- specific indicators tied to its immunization policy and programmatic actions. The resource map framework describes in detail the flow of resources and expenditures and how they are used within a health system, as Figure 6 shows.

Figure 6: Flow and Uses of Resources in a Health System

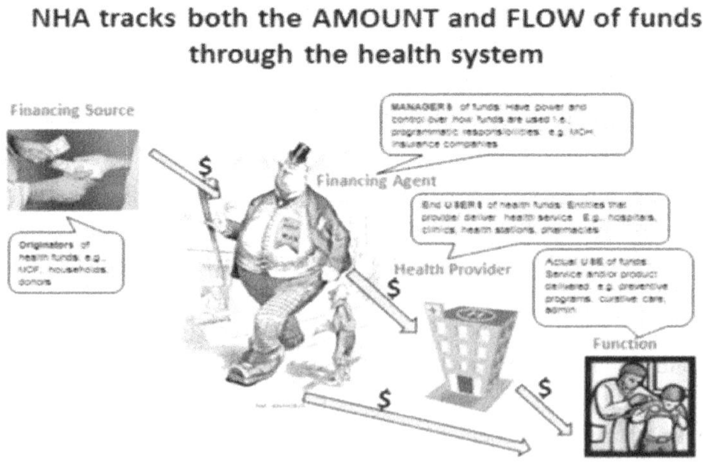

NHA tracks both the AMOUNT and FLOW of funds through the health system

Source: MOH&SW (2013)

When assessing health care strategies and policies, there is generally a lack of information on the management and the political process involved. The methodological approach includes the strategy of resource mapping to organize and compile data that focus not only on the flow and use of resources, but also on questions of power, relationships, processes and accountability in the EPI. Such questions include (MOH&SW 2013):Where does the money come from?

- Who manages and organises these funds?
- Where do these funds go?
- What goods and services are produced or bought by these funds?
- Who uses those goods and services?
- On which types of diseases or health services are these funds utilized?
- How these funds are distributed across the country?

Tools

1. Assessment of tools

The section assesses and reviews tools identified from the literature with a view to selecting the most suitable tools to be used for the stakeholder analysis and answering the above questions in measuring the dimensions of efficiency and sustainability of the EPI.

PHR financing assessment of immunization services tool

The methodology of this tool was developed for four PHR country case studies (Kaddar et al 2000) namely, Bangladesh, Colombia, Ivory Coast and Morocco, making it suitable for use in a developing country like The Gambia. Apart from this, it has as its primary objective the improvement of the financial sustainability of national immunization programmes. The tool focuses on these components: valuation of the costs and financing of immunizations programmes, National Immunization Days (NIDs) and mop-up activities, funding by programme component, evaluation of the trends in funding amounts from local and external sources, analysis of vaccine supply, procurement and financing, analysis of the impact of the current financing strategies on utilization, coverage, and equity, evaluation of the costs of closing access gaps, increasing coverage, and introducing new vaccines and technologies. It also focuses on the determination of the gaps between estimation of needed and anticipated funding, estimation of the potential for increasing local resource mobilization and appropriate and efficient use of external funding, and identification of options for financing strategies for the next multi-year timeframe.

The tool offers a checklist and tables that guide the user through information gathering, estimating current costs and financing, and developing a five-year plan. It will help managers to document the costs and financing status and related issues, and analyze trends in costing and financing, and effectively integrate data collection, analysis, planning, and decision-making. Programme managers and donors can develop policies to ensure the financial sustainability of the existing programme and plan improvements in terms of expanding coverage and adding new vaccines and technologies.

On the basis of the methodology, Kaddar et al, 2001 used the following framework (Table 7) to analyse data in the four country case studies.

Table 7: Data analysis framework

Sources of Financing	**Type of costs**	
	Capital Costs	**Recurrent Costs**
Internal		
External		

This framework (Kaddar et al, 2001) presents an organisation of financing data for analysis. It shows whether internal sources (e.g. central government, local government, health insurance and private sector) are being used for financing capital and recurrent costs. It also shows how external sources (donors, development banks, and international organisations) support has been targeted or used. Managers and donors can use this information to evaluate the roles and responsibilities of the government, NGOs, the private sector, and international donors in financing the NIP. Sustainability for the long- term is strengthened by a country's ability to finance recurrent costs, and to devote external funding to investment costs, for instance, assistance in introducing new vaccines and purchase of cold chain equipment (e.g. Kaddar et al, 2001).

The WHO common assessment tool for immunization services

The Common Assessment Tool (CAT) for Immunization Services describes the methodology for assessing immunization services in the wider context of the health system. Using the CAT should increase one's knowledge of the current and potential capacity of the health system and the individual programme, and system competencies that are necessary to improve performance. Assessments carried out using the CAT can also provide the information needed to develop or update national plans and prepare proposals for securing the support of development partners.

The method of the tool is based on the qualitative approach, which aims to find more than just facts and figures. It is built on collecting and analysing data about immunisation services, the health system, and the external environment. Data is collected for each of these components at the national, sub-national and service delivery levels. Data collection guides are used for gathering information. These give people at the sub-national and service delivery levels more opportunity to talk about what they consider the key issues to be, and what their possible solutions are.

One can use the methodology of the tool for planning an immunization programme to:

- Increase the accessibility and use of routine immunization services, especially for people who are not currently reached
- Improve the quality of immunization services
- Introduce new vaccines and new technologies
- Support increased financing for immunization services
- Support health system development.

The assessment methodology is based on the four principles below:

1. Performance is the measure of quality, efficiency, and the impact of immunization services.
2. Initially, one will investigate performance problems at the service delivery level and track those that do not have local causes through the system until one finds their origin.
3. Change can only take place if the people who know what the problems are, and who will make the recommendations, are engaged in identifying the problems.
4. The health system and the external environment strongly influence who is immunised and how immunization is provided, so the assessment methodology examines both the health system and the environment. Immunisation is just one of the health services the health system provides, so you should consider it as operating on its own. The strengths and weaknesses of immunisation services will have implications for the health system, and changes to one will affect the other.

Global alliance for vaccination and immunization (GAVI) tools

GAVI commissioned a paper (Levine et al 2001) entitled Financial Immunisation of Childhood Immunisation: Issues and Options that provides several frameworks for measuring the financial sustainability of immunization. The paper looks at financial sustainability as part of good management of immunization programmes, and the components of financial sustainability as facets that overlap with sound programme management. The paper identifies nine dimensions of financial sustainability of an immunization system that are considered under the categories of efficiency in the supply chain and appropriate funding structure.

The paper (Levine et al 2001) presents a set of criteria to judge potential indicators for measuring the financial sustainability of immunization. These criteria are validity and reliability, availability of data, relevance to workers/ ease of explanation, applicability to varied country contexts, and correspondence to high-priority policies and/or programmatic actions. On the basis of these criteria and the nine dimensions of financial sustainability of immunization systems, Levine et al developed several indicators (see chapter 3, section 3.4) that can be used by countries for measuring the financial sustainability of their immunization programmes.

However, the variations across countries and programmes pose a challenge to those countries seeking to establish uniform indicators and to set targets towards financial sustainability. There is little consistency in the availability of data from country to country, or in the priority that should be accorded to specific policy and programmatic actions in the long-term search for financial sustainability. Also, there are wide differences across countries and programmes in the extent in which efficiency measures can contribute to financial sustainability. To address this challenge, a core set of indicators of financial sustainability that would require information that is available in the country, together with country-specific indicators were selected for the study. Furthermore, this exercise of selecting indicators was conducted in a participatory manner involving major stakeholders. Other key indicators for immunization assessment.

There are other sets of indicators for the assessment of immunization services shown by the literature. The report of a meeting entitled Assessment of Immunization Services and Coordination of GAVI Activities at Country Level (WHO, 2000) provides several indicators for immunization assessment guidelines under these categories: immunization service delivery, immunization safety, logistics, vaccine supply and quality, advocacy and communication, surveillance, finance, and new vaccines/innovation. Another report of a meeting called Immunisation Finance Sustainability Plans, International Conference Centre Geneva, 4th-6th June 2001 (WHO, 2001) outlines several potential indicators for measuring financial sustainability. The group of participants at this conference used the list of indicators from the paper prepared for GAVI by Levine et al (2001) as a template in considering two levels of indicators.

2. Overview of tools

When looked at in terms of their appropriateness to the goals, objectives and questions of the study both the FI tool and Common Assessment tool for immunization services prove to be useful for measuring the component of funding sustainability, but insufficient with regard to questions on other aspects of sustainability of immunizations. Specifically, they are inadequate for answering the questions of where additional resources should be directed, and how adding vaccines would affect the infrastructure and sustainability of the programme. These are issues that must be considered in looking at programme efficiency and sustainability.

Furthermore, while the framework for analysis that the FI tool provides may be useful in providing information that can be used by stakeholders in financing the EPI (It shows whether internal sources---central government, local government, health insurance, private sector, etc. are being used for financing capital and recurrent costs. It also shows how external sources---donors, development banks, and international organisations support has been targeted). It lacks sufficient information on issues such as control of financing (GAVI funds controlled by Govt.?), commitment of financing (short-term, long-term, fixed-term/open-ended?), reliability of funder, and conditions of funding. Also, it considers costs as capital or recurrent costs. All costs should be shown as recurrent for purposes of assessing the sustainability of an ongoing programme (e.g. capital goods are replacements not investments----if a vehicle needs to be replaced every 5 years it costs $2000 per year, not $10, 000 every 10 years)

However, all the sets of indicators of financial sustainability contained in both tools are relevant and were considered for possible adoption for the study. To address these issues of sustainability sufficiently and answer the questions of the study, a Stakeholder Analysis questionnaire (Schmeer 1999) has been identified from the literature for adoption. As indicated, the stakeholder analysis uses a process of systematically gathering and analysing qualitative information from stakeholders (actors- persons or organisations- who have a vested interest in a policy that is being promoted) to determine whose interests should be taken into account when developing and/or implementing a policy or programme. Selected indicators of financial sustainability in the FI and Common Assessment tools, together with country-specific ones, are incorporated in the Stakeholder Analysis questionnaire. Also, a Resource Map questionnaire has been developed to complement the Stakeholder Analysis tool. The resource map framework describes in detail the flow of resources and expenditures and how they are used within a system on the basis of the National Health Accounts methodology outlined in detail in chapter 5. The methodologies of developing and applying these tools are described in detail in chapters 9 and 10. The following section presents a description of the tools.

3. Description of the tools

Stakeholder analysis questionnaire

This tool consists of four sections focusing on several stakeholder information or characteristics. Based on a review of the literature and PHR country experiences (Schmeer, 2001) these characteristics have been identified as the most important because:

i. Stakeholder knowledge is important in identifying stakeholders who oppose the issue of whether to use additional resources for improving the EPI infrastructure and not for introducing new vaccines due to misunderstanding or lack of communication
ii. The stakeholder's position on the issue of whether to use additional resources for improving the EPI infrastructure and not for introducing new vaccines is crucial to whether or not he/she will block its implementation.

As mentioned, in addition the tool incorporates qualitative statements of indicators (Table 8) that provide a basis for measuring progress towards the financial sustainability of the EPI. These statements include those focusing on the issues of providing reliable and sufficient funding for the EPI, as well as statements dealing with improvement in the supply chain, based on a broad definition of financial sustainability (Levine et al, 2001). These indicators developed by Levine et al (2001) can be used by countries for measuring the sustainability of their immunization programmes.

Table 8: Levine et al indicators of financial sustainability of immunisation programmes

A. Efficiency in the supply chain

A1. *Sustained demand and reduced barrier to access:*

⇒ Identifying levels of existing knowledge of and demand for immunization
⇒ Sponsoring public information and social mobilization programmes
⇒ Managing public information
⇒ Conducting situational analysis to identify critical barriers
⇒ Developing targeted programmes to reduce barriers (new delivery strategies
⇒ through public or private sectors

A2. *Efficient vaccine procurement*

⇒ Using international procurement mechanisms

A3. *Efficient immunization services*

⇒ Systematically assessing sources of waste
⇒ Developing and implementing targeted programmes to reduce waste, with
⇒ quantitative endpoints
⇒ Exploring potential for outsourcing support functions

B. Reliable and sufficient resources

B1. *Steady and sufficient funding for vaccines*
⇒ Forecasting requirements accurately
⇒ Developing line-item in national budgets
⇒ Fostering political action/or legal mandate for baseline funding levels

B2. *Steady and sufficient funding for labour and other non-vaccine recurrent costs*
⇒ Estimating total programme costs
⇒ Promoting allocation of resources on the basis of cost-effectiveness and public finance principles
⇒ Developing line-item in national budgets
⇒ Fostering political and/or legal mandate for baseline funding levels
⇒ Determining potential for private sector partnerships
⇒ Determining potential for insurance coverage of immunization

B3. *Steady and sufficient funding for investments (capital costs)*
⇒ Putting aside funds annually, based on amortisation schedule
⇒ Protecting investments for immunisation programme in national budgets

B4. *Stable resource flow to service delivery points*
⇒ Creating complete and accurate sub-national plans
⇒ Developing line items in sub-national budgets 146
⇒ Earmarking funds and establishing performance targets for sub-national entities

B5. *Balanced public-private financing*
⇒ Assessing current patterns of use and financing
⇒ Identifying barriers to greater private sector participation and low-cost ways to overcome them

B6. *Effective mobilization and management of supplementary, external resources and log-term financing*

⇒ Demonstrating increasing national commitment by adopting efficiency measures and assuring consistent relative domestic contributions

⇒ Demonstrating commitment to "additionality" (Extent to which a new item or action adds to the existing item or actions, without replacing any of them, and results in increasing the total)

⇒ Coordinating support, and utilising financial planning tools

⇒ Negotiating long-term financing (Levine et al 2001)

The tool starts with an introductory section that the interviewer can read to the stakeholder. It includes mostly open-ended questions requiring the stakeholder to provide more than a simple "Yes" or "No" answer. Indirect questions are included wherever possible to prevent unreliable answers. Where necessary, several questions are posed in order to obtain information on one characteristic or statement of indicator. Also, tables for summarising stakeholders' ratings on the indicators are included.

4. Resource map questionnaire

This questionnaire is divided into three categories of organisational roles on the provision of resources (a source of support or aid; can be financial, technological, political, and other (Webster, 1984) for EPI-related activities based on the NHA methodology described in chapter 5:

1. Sources of finance---- organisations or persons providing resources for EPI-related activities;
2. Financing Intermediaries---- organisations or persons through which resources are channelled to service providers;
3. Providers---- service providers who receive resources from financing intermediaries, or directly from financing sources for carrying out EPI-related activities.

Questions under the sources of finance category focus on expenditures which organisations make within a five- year period, the EPI-related activities for which organisations provide resources and the amounts (quantities) spent on each activity. For the financing intermediary's category, the focus of the questions is on resources that are channelled through organisations in a year and the amounts, procedures for securing more needed resources, where funds go from organisations and how funds are used, and decision-making about the movement and use of funds. Questions under the provider's category centre on sources of resources used for EPI-related activities, the specific functions for which funds are used, decision-making about the use of funds, and coverage for each vaccine. In addition, questions focus on opinions about present and potential problems, funding levels, the best use of additional resources, and how to improve immunization services.

There is an introductory section that the interviewer can read to the respondent. The tool includes mostly open-ended questions, a few structured questions, and a list of EPI-related activities to enable respondents to indicate the EPI-related activities for which their organisations provide resources.

Summary

We have in this chapter considered the case study methodological approach including its rationale, the aim, objectives and questions of the study, its conceptual framework, and its structure, including the tools and their assessment and description. The methodological approach provided theoretical foundation for understanding which method, set of methods or best practices can be applied to assessing the sustainability of immunisation programme in the Gambia, specifically dealing with the question of whether to use the limited resources to introduce new vaccines, or rather to use such resources for improving the EPI infrastructure. It allowed for the systematic study of methods that can be applied within the EPI, and the analysis of the principles of methods, rules, and postulates used by the discipline. Chapters 9 and 10 that follow describe how this methodological approach was developed and applied mainly in terms of the stakeholder analysis and resource map tools. We begin with the development and application of the stakeholder analysis tool.

9

The Methodology of Developing and Applying the Stakeholder analysis tool

The Stakeholder Analysis methodology comprised three stages (Schmeer, 1999). The first stage focused on the identification of groups and individuals relevant to immunization financing and sustainability. The second stage dealt with the assessment of the political resources of relevant groups and individuals and their roles in the political structures to determine their relative power for the financing and sustainability of the immunization programme. The third stage concentrated on evaluating their present position on the financing and sustainability of the programme, including their underlying interests and the intensity of their commitment. This analytical task was conducted by the researchers (the writer as principal researcher and a trained research assistant) who organised the qualitative data obtained for these assessments, searched for themes, items and patterns, validated the understanding obtained and interrelated various themes to provide a comprehensive structure to the data. The following sections describe in detail these steps.

5. Identification of groups and individuals relevant to immunization sustainability

Two distinct modes of analysis were combined: interest group analysis and bureaucratic politics analysis. The former analysis consisted of understanding those social groups that are seeking to press the government in a particular direction, including private business and non-governmental organizations. The latter analysis focused on the competition between the government and individuals. Such stakeholders relevant to the immunization programme include both players outside and inside government. The analysis also included consideration of the activities of international agencies, like the World Bank, UNICEF and the World Health Organisation. The following kinds of interest groups were involved in the analysis:

- Producer Groups---health sector workers and their unions, and international equipment and vaccine manufacturers.
- Bureaucratic Groups-----bureaucratic organisations related to immunisation (e.g. Department of State for Health and Social Welfare and Department of State for Finance & Economic Affairs)
- Economic Groups--- industries related to immunizations (e.g. vaccine dealers), and workers in EPI.
- Health development Groups----bilateral aid agencies, international health organizations, multilateral development banks, non-governmental organizations.

For the examination of bureaucratic groups, the following government actors in addition to the Department of State for Health & Social Welfare (DOSH&SW) were involved in the political analysis:

- Department of State for Finance and Economic Affairs- especially in terms of changes in the financing of immunization or changes in the DOSH&SW's budget, and calculation about overall economic growth, among other things.
- Local and Area Councils--in terms of decentralization of health services, including immunization services.
- Department of State for Education---for policies that affect health, nursing, public health and medical schools
- Department of State for Trade, Employment and Industry- for policies on vaccines, equipment and human resources.

The compilation of the list of stakeholders was guided by these questions: Who cares about immunization financing and sustainability? Who is likely to act, or could be convinced to act? Who has the potential to influence the outcome? Who is likely to be affected by the consequences of the reforms on immunization financing, both positively and negatively?

6. Assessment of the political resources of relevant groups and individuals and their roles in the political structures

The power and influence of each of the players listed above (the groups and individuals who are relevant to immunisation financing and sustainability) were estimated. An assessment of the following for each player was conducted:

- The player's political resources and place in the political system, which determine the political capacity to influence policy decisions
- The player's interests, position, alliances and commitment, which will influence how the player's resources, and how much of those resources will be used in improving the financing and sustainability of the EPI.

The political resources that were concentrated on included tangible resources like money, organization, equipment and offices, and how they affect a group's ability to influence decisions on the financing of immunisation. The political resources also included intangibles, such as information on immunisation and related problems, relevant substantive expertise, which allows the group to develop a position, group alliances and the group's visibility and legitimacy.

7. Evaluation of stakeholders' present position on the financing and sustainability of the EPI.

Assessment of how each group's views and position on immunization financing and sustainability focused, first, on the group's interests, as this may determine the political position of the group on the issue of whether to use additional resources for improving the EPI infrastructure and funding and not for introducing new vaccines. Then the positions that the players have taken publicly were examined, and the intensity of each group's current position on the issue described.

These were the three stages of the case study methodology of the stakeholder analysis. These methods are further described in the following discussion of the methodology of developing and applying the stakeholder analysis tool. This consists of several steps for identifying information sources, conducting interviews and creating tools from generic frameworks. The steps are described as follows:

Selecting stakeholders

First, the researcher met with the health economist at the Medical Research Council (MRC) and the Manager and staff of the EPI Unit, Department of State for Health & Social Welfare, to identify potential stakeholders from sectors such as donor organisations. The discussion focused on persons or organisations that might be related to or affected by the issue of financial sustainability of the EPI and have a direct interest in the issue of whether to use additional resources for improving the EPI infrastructure and funding and not for introducing new vaccines and the ability to influence decisions on the issue. With the help of the experts and based on guidelines for conducting a stakeholder analysis (Schmeer 1999) the researcher defined the list of stakeholders to be interviewed for the pre-test. The initial list consisted of the Head of a divisional health team, the Medical Officer and Matron in-charge of the polyclinic under the Royal Victoria Teaching Hospital, the MCH and IEC Coordinators in the Department of State for Health & Social Welfare, the Manager of the CISP-Italian Fund, and the Registrar, Gambia Nurses and Midwives Council.

To be selected stakeholders:

1. Had to have a professional or socially responsible association to the issue of immunization financing and sustainability;
2. Were likely to act, or could be convinced to act;
3. Must have had the potential to influence the outcome;
4. Were likely to be affected by the consequences of any potential the reforms on immunization financing, both positively and negatively

Although 'users' may be affected by supply and delivery of immunisation, they were excluded mainly because they (in this case mothers and their children), as Schmeer (1999) points out, are unlikely to be directly related to the specifics of financing and the particular issue under debate [of whether additional resources should be directed toward improving the EPI infrastructure and funding and not for introducing new vaccines]. All those eligible were included in the study, including donors.

Developing questions

Second, using the guidelines, the researcher reviewed and adopted the stakeholder characteristics and definitions (Schmeer 1999): interests, alliances, resources, leadership and stakeholder's agreement or disagreement on the indicators of financial sustainability.

Once the stakeholder characteristics and terms had been defined, a stakeholder analysis table was created based on the generic one provided in the guidelines by (Schmeer 1999). The table covered the stakeholder characteristics such as alliance, resources and leadership.

Developing format of the tool

Third, a standard questionnaire was developed from the generic tool provided in the literature (Schmeer 1999). The most important aim of such a development is to explore a framework for including qualitative statements of indicators that provide a basis for measuring progress towards the financial sustainability of the EPI in a stakeholder analysis tool.

Having decided to use a stakeholder analysis process and indicators of financial sustainability to achieve the objectives, it was necessary to consider which indicators to use. As mentioned, in the Gambia the period beginning 1979 when the Expanded Programme on Immunization was launched to 1994 was characterised by the mobilization of substantial resources, due to the highest priority afforded the EPI by external donors, such as the WHO, USAID, UNICEF and the Italian Government. During this period, the EPI has steadily increased coverage to 80% of the fully immunized child less than one year of age (Gambia EPI Review 2001).

However, in 1994 after the coup this situation changed significantly with progressive disengagement of many partners of the government. Although the Government allocated a high proportion of funds to the programme and the ADB and UNICEF provided substantial support to address the shortage of funds, there was a diminution in the annual total financing, including funds provided by the ADB and UNICEF. This decrease in donor contribution was also due to the high priority given to the NIDs. Since 1999, there has been a renewal of EPI financing through the efforts of the government, EDF, MRC, WHO and UNICEF, ADB and Area Councils (Kodjo et al, 2001), but despite such efforts the financial situation of the programme remains bleak, resulting in declines in immunization coverage, uncertainty of vaccine supply, aging cold chain equipment, interruption of outreach services due to lack of vaccines or transportation, high vaccine wastage rates, among other problems (Gambia EPI Review 2001).

Thus, these issues of instability in the EPI seem relevant for this study because they are of great importance for the sustainability of the EPI especially in terms of the government's ability to sufficiently finance the EPI and introduce new vaccines. Compared to other indicators of financial sustainability of the EPI identified in the literature which have a narrower focus, the set of indicators of financial sustainability selected for the study (Levine, 2001) encompass these broader, more practical aspects of financial sustainability of the EPI. As explained previously, these indicators are considered under dimensions of financial sustainability of immunization systems of low costs through efficiency in the supply chain and reliable and sufficient financing through appropriate funding structure. Keyed to these dimensions are actions (indicators) that the government can take to introduce or strengthen specific immunization policies, and can enhance programming management in certain ways. These are actions that the government will find useful in putting together its plan for financial sustainability under the GAVI mechanism.

This process of selecting indicators involved consultations with members of the research team including the health economist at MRC and the manager and staff of the EPI, and review of the relevant literature.

Development of Interview Protocol

Fourth, the principal researcher, with the help of the research assistant developed the interview protocol to be followed in the interview process, and the procedure for analysing the data. To ensure objectivity and consistency, the following protocol was used:

- The principal researcher and one trained research assistant should make up the interview team
- Both interviewers should take notes, with the Principal researcher leading the interview
- Interviews should also be recorded
- Questions should not be asked more than twice
- Where necessary, probing questions should be used such as: "You said that you would like to see the EPI infrastructure improved before any new vaccine is introduced?"
- Immediately following the interviews, interviewers should mark the tapes for easy identification

To address ethical issues, the principal researcher firstly applied to both the South Bank University Ethics Committee and the Gambia Government/MRC Ethics Committee for permission to conduct the study. The study proposal and outline including the questionnaires were made available to the appropriate authorities for review, and permissions were granted. The letters of approval were distributed for permission to carry out the study in the Gambia and to use the appropriate records and facilities the study demanded.

Pre-test

Fifth, a pre-test was conducted by interviewing the stakeholders listed above. The main purpose of the pre-testing was to ensure validity. The pre-test was conducted to determine the following:

Research procedure

- Availability of the study population
- Acceptability of the methods used to establish contact with the study population
- Acceptability of the questions asked
- Willingness of the respondents to answer the questions and collaborate

with the study
- Interviewers successfully adhered to the interview protocol

Data-collection tools
- The interviewee understands the questions
- Answers provide the information required
- The interview does not take more than two hours
- Whether there is any need to revise the format or presentation of questionnaires

Analysing the stakeholder table

The stakeholder table was analysed as follows:

Developing the framework

For this analysis, the stakeholders are divided into three groups:

⇒ Group 1 – those who have leadership and high power (Level 3)

⇒ Group 2 – those who have leadership and medium power (Level 2)

⇒ Group 3 – those who do not have leadership but have high to medium power (Level 2 or 3).

This analytic framework is based on the premise that those with leadership and power will be most able to affect policy implementation. Once the stakeholder table was completed, the information was "analysed." Such an analysis focused on comparing information and developing conclusions about the stakeholders' relative importance, knowledge, interests, positions, and possible allies regarding the issue in question: whether to use additional resources for improving the EPI infrastructure and funding and not for introducing new vaccines. From the information in the stakeholder table, the researchers concluded the following:
- Who the most important stakeholders are (from a power and leadership analysis);
- What the stakeholders' knowledge of the issue of whether to use additional resources for improving the EPI infrastructure and funding and not for introducing new vaccines is;
- What the stakeholders' positions on this specific issue are;
- What indicators of financial sustainability stakeholders agree or disagree on.
- What the stakeholders see as possible advantages or disadvantages of the issue of whether to use additional resources for improving the EPI infra-

structure and funding and not for introducing new vaccines (interest analysis); and

- Which stakeholders might form alliances

The specific steps for developing these five analyses are detailed below:

Carrying out power and leadership analysis

Although the intent in prioritizing the stakeholder list for the pre-test was to select only those stakeholders with power and leadership, the first analysis is designed to use the information from the table to further prioritize the stakeholders within the selected group interviewed. This second prioritization, based on actual data and a more select group, allows policy makers and managers to focus resources on addressing the concerns of the most important of the priority stakeholders. The "importance" of stakeholders is defined here as their ability to affect the implementation of the idea of putting more resources into the EPI in order to improve efficiency in the supply chain and reliable and sufficient funding and not to introduce new vaccines. Since power and leadership are the characteristics that determine a stakeholder's ability to affect or block the implementation of the idea of putting more resources into the EPI in order to improve efficiency in the supply chain and reliable and sufficient funding and not to introduce new vaccines, these two characteristics are the basis for the first "importance" analysis. Power: quantity of resources and ability to mobilize those resources for or against the idea of putting more resources into the EPI in order to improve efficiency in the supply chain and reliable and sufficient funding and not to introduce new vaccines. Leadership: a willingness to initiate, convoke, or lead an action for or against the idea of putting more resources into the EPI in order to improve efficiency in the supply chain and reliable and sufficient funding and not to introduce new vaccines.

The stakeholders making up these three groups were identified by organization rather than by name in order to preserve their anonymity. Each of the three groups has a name (this is simply group 1, 2, or 3).

Analysing knowledge data

The stakeholders' level of knowledge related to the policy also is often of interest to policy makers and managers. This level of knowledge was presented as a general conclusion, as it is similar for the majority of the stakeholders, and the stakeholders were also divided by their level of knowledge: 3, 2, or 1. the latter option is useful for targeting a communication strategy for a specific group of stakeholders, namely those with the lowest knowledge of the policy. These stakeholders would appear in Group 1 for knowledge level. The information found in the knowledge data was crossed with the power/leadership analysis to highlight the importance of the stakeholders with a low knowledge level. This cross-analysis would result in an even smaller priority group for targeting communication strategies. The knowledge data was also cross- referenced with the position of the stakeholders to determine if those opposed to the policy had a consistently low level of knowledge. If so, this would indicate to the policy maker or manager promoting this policy that communicating or advocating the objectives and basic tenets of the policy could reduce the opposition.

Analysing stakeholders' positions

In analysing the position information from the table, the following aspects were determined:

- Total number of supporters
- Importance of supporters (cross-reference with power/leadership analysis)
- Knowledge of supporters (cross-reference with knowledge data)
- Advantages and disadvantages of policy implementation to the supporters (cross-reference with interest data)
- Knowledge of whether these supporters are internal or external to the organization (DOSH&SW) developing EPI policy (cross-reference with the internal/ external classification)
- Support "clusters" – stakeholders in the same sector who support the idea of putting more resources into the EPI in order to improve efficiency in the supply chain and reliable and sufficient funding and not to introduce new vaccines (cross-reference with organization information)
- Total number of opponents
- Importance of opponents (cross-reference with power/leadership analysis)
- Knowledge of opponents (cross-reference with knowledge data)
- Advantages and disadvantages of implementation of the idea of using additional resources for improving the EPI infrastructure and funding and not for introducing new vaccines to the opponents (cross-reference with interest data)
- Knowledge of whether these opponents are internal or external to the organization (DOSH&SW) developing EPI policy (cross-reference with the internal/external classification)
- Opposition "clusters" – stakeholders in the same sector who oppose the idea of putting more resources into the EPI in order to improve efficiency in the supply chain and reliable and sufficient funding and not to intro-

duce new vaccines (cross-reference with organization information)

- Neutral stakeholders, their importance, knowledge, and interests. The researchers identified such conclusions directly from the stakeholder table.

Analysing indicator data

The indicator data were used in connection with other analyses as well as alone as general conclusions. In cross-referencing the indicator data, the stakeholder's agreement and/or disagreement with the indicators of financial sustainability were used with other data to emphasize the importance of the indicators. For example, the indicator data were cross-referenced with the power/ leadership data to indicate what the most important stakeholders consider to be the most useful indicators, indicators that they see as lacking in value in the Gambian context, and the extent to which the actions have been taken by the government.

Analysing interest data

The interest data were also used in conjunction with other analyses as well as alone as general conclusions. In cross-referencing the interest data, the policy implementation advantages and disadvantages the stakeholders identified were used with other data to explain the positions of the stakeholders or to emphasize their knowledge of the issue of whether to use additional resources for improving the EPI infrastructure and funding and not for introducing new vaccines policy (i.e., if irrelevant advantages and disadvantages were identified, it may represent a misunderstanding of the issue). The interest data were also cross-referenced with the power/leadership data to indicate what the most important stakeholders may have to lose or gain from implementation of the idea of putting more resources into the EPI in order to improve efficiency in the supply chain and reliable and sufficient funding and not to introduce new vaccines.

Analysing alliances

Possible stakeholder alliances were also identified from the table information. The alliances were identified in two ways: (1) by referring to the stakeholder table to see if stakeholders mentioned organizations that they would work with to demonstrate for or against the idea of using additional resources for improving the EPI infrastructure and funding and not for introducing new vaccines or (2) by referring to the position "clusters" (the stakeholders with similar positions and within the same organization or sub-sector). The alliance information was cross-referenced with the position data to identify those alliances that may be potential sources of support, as well as those that may work together to oppose the idea of putting more resources into the EPI in order to improve efficiency in the supply chain and reliable and sufficient funding and not to introduce new vaccines. The researchers suggested the development of specific strategies based on these key alliances, either to reinforce a potentially supportive alliance or to separate a potentially threatening alliance, or other specific strategies. The alliance data were also cross-referenced with the power/leadership analysis results to highlight those alliances that were potentially the most supportive or threatening to the implementation of the idea of putting more resources into the EPI in order to improve efficiency in the supply chain and reliable and sufficient funding and not to introduce new vaccines.

Adopting the information transfer reference chart

Sixth, a final tool, the information transfer reference chart was adopted from the Guidelines. The purposes of this tool were (1) to help the research team in transferring the information from the questionnaire to the stakeholder table and (2) to provide a means of checking that all the stakeholder characteristics are included in the interview questionnaire.

Summary

This chapter has described the methodology of developing and applying the stakeholder analysis tool. There are three distinct steps in the development and application process, including the development of the tool, identification of information sources, developing questions and analyzing stakeholder data. The following chapter deals with the development and application of the complementary resource map tool.

10

Methodology of Developing and Applying the Resource Map tool

A comprehensive estimation of the total amount of resources available to the EPI might firstly be based on funds available for the EPI from the Gambia's Department of State for Finance & Economic Affairs, and fee income. In a developing country like The Gambia, where private expenditures make 80% of total health expenditure, it is necessary to obtain projections of resources coming from out-of-pocket expenditures, various forms of health insurance, private firms and voluntary organisations. As well as providing an estimate of the amount of money available for immunisation, resource projections will also inform decisions about priorities for public spending. The preparation of national accounts, which relates sources and uses of funds, as we have seen especially in chapter 5, is particularly useful in such estimation (Cassels, 1997). This chapter firstly outlines a three-phase process of developing and applying the resource map tool.

Three-Phase Process

Drawing both on the traditional National Health Accounts (NHA) methodology, a three-phase process was used involving: 1) the identification of information sources; 2) data collection; and 3) analysis and dissemination of results.

Phase One: Identification and inventory of information sources

Before data collection was begun, an exhaustive inventory of public and private sector organizations and agencies involved in EPI-related activities was made. First, however, a definition of what constitutes "EPI related activities" was established in order to consistently disaggregate EPI expenditures from other expenditures. Both the definition and inventory processes involved consultations and brainstorming with the National Immunisation Programme and other local expert groups.

The application of the NHA framework to the EPI in The Gambia

Definition of EPI expenditures

For this project, we define EPI expenditures as those that have a direct impact on the provision of EPI services. A list of the types of activities that might fall under EPI-related activities was discussed with on-site staff in the Gambia; only they will be able to accurately determine what definition makes sense in the local context. In addition, interviews with local experts and government officials were conducted to determine the appropriate desegregation of funds applied to multiple end uses. The list is shown in Table 9.

Table 9: EPI-related activities

- Research and evaluation
- Supplementary immunization
- Monitoring and supervision
- Human resource development
- Vaccine supply and quality
- Cold chain and logistics
- Social mobilization
- Programme management
- Injection safety
- Disease control/surveillance
- Disease eradication

Definition of EPI-related activities

Given the complexity of the data collection in this study and the availability of data, among other things, the researcher focused exclusively on expenditures that are directly EPI-related. Expenditures that have only an indirect relationship to EPI work, such as school fees, were, as already mentioned, not considered in this activity.

Inventory of entities involved in EPI-related activities

Next, an exhaustive inventory of public and private sector organisations and agencies involved in EPI-related activities was made. These organizations were categorized as sources of financing, financing intermediaries, and service providers based on the NHA classification of flows of funds, as outlined below. These sources are organised, intermediaries, and end users by whether they are in the public or private sector. However, funds may of course flow between the public and the private sectors.

Categorization of public sector entities involved in EPI-related activities

Sources of financing

- Department of State for Finance & Economic Affairs

Financing intermediary

- Department of State for Health & Social Welfare

Providers

- Public health facilities (primary, secondary, and tertiary)

Categorization of private sector entities involved in EPI-related Activities

Sources of financing

- International donors
- NGOs
- Procurement companies/manufacturers
- Micro-finance institutions

Providers

- Private/NGO health facilities (primary, secondary and tertiary)
- Clubs/Associations
- Churches

* The DOSH&SW is the main financing intermediary

Inventory of data sources

After creating an inventory of the organisations involved in EPI-related activities, an inventory of information sources was made. Potential information sources used are listed below:

Potential information sources

Information on sources of financing

- published financial reports from bilateral donor organisations
- published financial reports from the UN and other multilateral agencies
- surveys sent to donor organisations
- interviews with donor organisations
- national and local government budgets
- interviews with staff of the DOSF&EA and other relevant government departments
- interviews with staff at relevant NGOs

Information on financing intermediary

- national and local government budgets
- DOSH&SW budgets
- interviews with staff at relevant government departments
- interviews with staff of NGOs

Information on providers

- interviews with hospital and clinic personnel
- discussions with experts in the field
- records of providers
- interviews with advocacy groups

Phase Two: Data collection activities

This section outlines the steps that were followed to obtain expenditure data in The Gambia. The Gambia data was collected to give the true picture of the health financing

Obtaining data on expenditures for EPI-related programmes from bilateral and multilateral aid organisations, and comparing with country-reported receipt of bilateral funding

Under the NHA activity, reports on donor expenditures are being requested both from the donor agencies and from the Gambian government. The researchers (the writer and a trained research assistant) focused on EPI-specific assistance. Significant double-checking was made to account for any differences between their reported amounts. As much detail as possible about the end uses of the funding was requested, and interviews with the representatives of donor agencies and government officials were held to ensure a thorough analysis.

Obtaining reports of government expenditures on EPI-related activities; reviewing these reports, and interviewing national and local officials

The research team (the writer as principal researcher and a trained research assistant) contacted the appropriate Departments of State in The Gambia to request information on national expenditures on EPI-related programmes. Determining government spending in the National Immunisation Programme is relatively straightforward. Government spending related to EPI work in other sectors (for instance, under education budgets, women's programmes, or social welfare programmes to improve immunisation coverage, as well as spending at the municipal or district level), requires more in-depth analysis. It is likely that officially reported expenditures would underestimate the total resources devoted to EPI-related work in the country. Interviews with national and local officials may be necessary to capture under-reported activities. In many cases, national and local officials will have to estimate the proportion of integrated programmes that should be considered EPI-related. Budgets were reviewed both to determine the amounts of EPI funding and to determine the particular agencies and organisations that are the recipients of such funding. These agencies were then contacted, to determine how the funding was actually spent in the field.

Estimation of primary, secondary, and tertiary health facility expenditures on EPI

The Gambia's Health Information unit of the Department of State for Health & Social Welfare collects monthly statistical reports on health facility utilization from the health divisions for outpatients and in-patients. Expenditures data are central, and data on revenues from all divisions, including clinics, etc, are provided through the Drug Revolving Fund (DRF) office. All these quantitative data were collected and analysed during the period of the study March-June 2004 for use in the resource map study (Tables 10 & 11 below). Also, where possible, the researchers collected data on-site from health facility records in the health facilities included in the study. This helped in determining how many individuals were immunized, the frequency of immunization visits, and the costs incurred. Also, where possible the researcher obtained facility-level data on the EPI expenditures and the use of resources through interviews with facility staff.

Estimation of NGOs' and private sector organizations' expenditures on EPI-related activities

NGOs are often able to provide highly differentiated, cost-effective services to groups of clients, and are relied upon by national governments to provide services the governments cannot provide. Unfortunately, reporting on private sector expenditures is not nearly as standardised or consistent as reporting on government expenditures.

Interviews were held with NGOs involved in EPI work, asking about funding and expenditures relating to the EPI. The data obtained in this manner was validated with data obtained from donors, discussions, and interviews with prominent NGOs and employers.

Phase Three: Organisation and presentation of data

To organise and present the data four matrices were constructed. Each chart was divided between public and private expenditures. The total cost was consistent or equal across all of the matrices:

Matrix 1 shows the flow of resources from funding sources to intermediaries.
Matrix 2 shows the flow of resources from intermediaries to providers.
Matrix 3 shows the flow of resources from intermediaries to functions,
(i.e. immunisation activities)
Matrix 4 shows the flow of resources from providers to functions.

Several corresponding basic sets of tables (Tables 11, 12, 13 & 14) are created to illustrate the financial flow of funds between financing sources, financing intermediaries, providers and functions. Information on EPI expenditures and uses of funds was obtained from top DOSH&SW officials, including EPI officials, officials of donor agencies at the central level, as well as from providers at divisional and facility levels.

Findings from the interviews and documentary analysis suggest that the majority of resources mobilised in the EPI do not just pass directly from the ultimate sources to their final uses, as Figure 7 shows. Most of the resources pass through one main financial intermediary, the Department of State for Health & Social Welfare (green colour), which in turn transfers resources on to the ultimate providers of care. For all sources of funding, money is transferred to mainly the DOSH, which manages and organises the funds. The major sources in the flow of funds for the EPI are donors and the Department of State for Finance and Economic Affairs. The direction of the flow of funds varies depending on its sources and the main intermediary, the DOSH&SW, which is funded by quite different sources.

Figure 7: Flow of Funds through Immunisation System

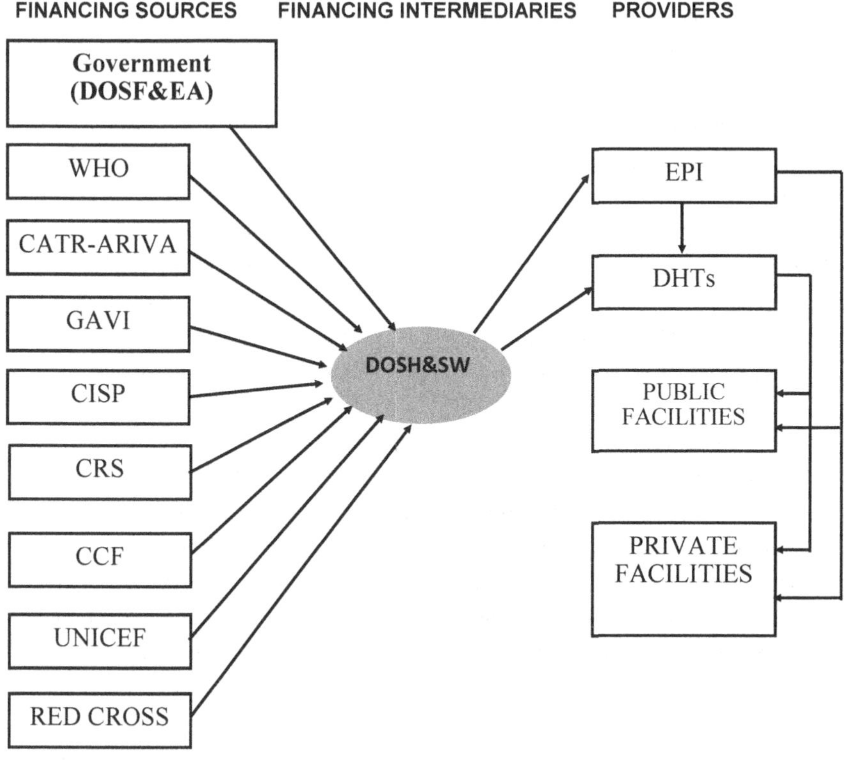

Source: Sarr 2005

The flow of resources from funding sources to intermediaries (Matrix 1) can be divided into two parts. Part 1 consists of the flow of funds from donors to the Department of State for Health & Social Welfare (DOSH&SW). Part 2 comprises funds from the Department of State for Finance and Economic Affairs (from general revenue sources) to the DOSH&SW. (Donors/ NGOs may however pass funds directly to the ultimate providers of immunization, mainly to the Divisional Health Teams (DHTs). This happens on very rare occasions, like emergencies). Resources flow from the DOSH&SW to providers, namely, the EPI, DHTs, public health facilities and a few private health facilities (Matrix 2). Also, resources flow from the DOSH&SW to functions at government and private facilities (Matrix 3). Finally, resources flow from providers to functions in both public and private facilities (Matrix 4)

Flow and uses of funds from financing sources to financing intermediary.

Table 10, Matrix 1 shows the flow of funds from financing sources to the main financing intermediary, the DOSH&SW, as generated from the questionnaire and documents of Government and donors, as well as from interviews with EPI staff. As Table 10 shows, in 2003 EPI costs amounted to $2, 364, 362.71. The most important portion of these costs is recurrent which represents 85% against 15% of capital expenditures. The low percentage of capital expenditures is partly due to the fact that most of such expenditures were carried out in previous years. 18% of the total amount of $2, 364, 362.71 was contributed by Government (Department of State for Finance &Economic Affairs (DOSF&EA), 13% by UNICEF, 7% by WHO, 0.87% by CATR (European Union Project), 1% by the Red Cross, 1% by CISP (Italian Fund), 0.10% by the Christian Children's Fund (CCF), 0.57% by MRC, 0.35% by the African Development Bank (ADB), 55% by the Global Alliance for Vaccines and Immunisation (GAVI), 0.07% by the Catholic Relief Services (CRS) and 3% by other donors. These figures show a higher percentage of expenditure by the donor community when compared to government's expenditure.

Table 11, Matrix 2 details the allocation of resources from the Financing Intermediary to EPI activities/functions: research and evaluation, supplementary immunisation, monitoring and supervision, human resource development, vaccine supply and quality, cold chain logistics, social mobilisation, programme management, injection safety, and disease control/surveillance. As can be seen, on average the highest amount of resources (64%) went to the activity of vaccine supply and quality. Relatively, there were few contributions to the other functions, particularly to the functions of research and evaluation (0.44%), monitoring and supervision (1%), human resource development (2%) and disease control/surveillance (0.72%). These figures show significant variation in the use of resources by EPI activity or function.

Table 10, Matrix 1: Financing sources to financing intermediary

Financing Sources	DOSH & SW	TOTAL %
GOVERNMENT (DoSF & EA)	418,040US$	18
UNICEF	302,224US$	13
WHO	162,028 US$	7
CATR	20,542 US$	0.87
RED CROSS	26,180 US$	1
CISP	29,907 US$	1
CCF	2,409 US$	0.10
MRC	13,464 US$	0.57
ADB	8,364 US$	0.35
GAVI	1,297,520 US$	55
CRS	1,647 US$	0.07
OTHER DONORS	82,037 US$	3
TOTAL	**2,364,363 US$**	100

Table 11, Matrix 2: Financing intermediary to function

Functions	DOSH & SW (US$)	TOTAL (%)
1. Research & Evaluation	10.431	0.44
2. Supplementary Immunization	74, 916	3
3. Monitoring & Supervision	27,180	1
4. Human Resource Dev	38,786	2
5. Vaccine Supply and quality	1,510,518	64
6. Cold Chain Logistics	89,134	4
7. Social Mobilisation	64,860	3
8. Programme Management	411,688	17
9. Injection Safety	119,830	5
10. Disease Control/Surveillance	17,020	0.72
Total	**2,364,363**	**100**

Source: Sarr (2005)

Flow and uses of funds from financing intermediary to providers

Table 12, Matrix 3 shows the quantity of resources from the financing intermediary allocated to the different providers of immunisation as generated from the questionnaire and interviews with DOSH&SW top officials and EPI staff and donors. The results detail the allocation of resources by facility and level of the EPI: central level (EPI Unit), divisional level (Divisional Health Teams), and facility (public and private hospitals, health centres, clinics and outreach stations) levels. Consistent with the volume of service delivery at the facility level, the health facilities used the most resources. On average 74% of the total EPI expenditure of $2,364, 362.71 allocated to service providers in 2003 went to public facilities and 10% went to private facilities. However, this shows the relatively higher weight of spending in public facilities when compared to spending in private facilities. The central level utilised 9% while the divisional level used 7%.

Flow and uses of funds from providers to functions

Table 13, Matrix 4 shows the amount of resources providers use to carry out each of the various EPI activities/functions. Again, it can be seen that most of the expenditure is utilised in facilities for vaccine supply and quality activities (85% and 14%), with private facilities receiving a relatively smaller share of the expenditure on this activity. Notably, there were no expenditures on research and evaluation in both public and private facilities. Also to be noted is not only the relatively small amounts of expenditures directed to other activities in private facilities, but also the absence of expenditure in private facilities on the activities of monitoring and supervision and programme management. The above sections have outlined the flow and uses of funds in the immunisation system. The following section will present a description of the procedures used in financing and using resources in the immunisation system, with regard to the three principal categories of actors within the system- financing sources, financing intermediary and providers.

Table 1 2, Matrix 3: Financing intermediary to providers

Providers	DOSH&SW	TOTAL (%)
Central (EPI)	208,375	9
Divisional (DHT)	165,050	7
Public Facilities	1,752,824	74
Private Facilities	237,414	10
Total	2,364,363	100

Table 13, Matrix 4: Providers to Functions

Function	Central (EPI)	Divisional (DHTs)	Public Facilities	Private Facilities	Total
Research & Evaluation	2,489 (24%)	7,242 (49%)	-	-	10,431
Supplementary Immunization	5,535 (7%)	17,500 (23%)	440,981 (59%)	7,782 (10%)	74,916
Monitoring & Supervision	12,727 (47%)	3.018 (11%)	11,436 (42%)	-	27,180
Human Resource Devel-	1,735 (4%)	10,677 (28%)	23,599 (61%)	2,775 (7%)	38,786
Vaccine Supply and quality	12,914 (1%)	4,045 (0.27)	1,280,001 (85%)	213,558 (14%)	1,510,518
Cold Chain Logistics	21,174 (24%)	21,427 (24%)	43,755 (49%)	2,778 (3%)	89,134
Social Mobilisation	508 (1%)	59,590 (92%)	4,081 (6%)	681 (1%)	64,160
Programme Management	141,389 (36%)	35,083 (9%)	235, 215 (57%)	-	411,688
Injection Safety	5, 597 (5%)	1, 734 (1%)	103,800 (87%)	8,698 (7%)	119,830
Disease Control/ Surveillance	4,307 (25%)	4,733 (28%)	6,839 (40%)	1,141 (17%)	17,020
Total	208,375 (9%)	165,050 (7%)	1, 752,824 (74%)	237,414 (10%)	2.364,363

Source: Sarr (2005)

Data Analysis

All quantitative data were analysed using Microsoft Excel statistical analysis. The researcher produced descriptive statistics like mean and standard deviations, frequency distributions and percentages.

Generally, qualitative data from interviews, documentary analysis and observations on aspects of the study, including the elements of finance and sustainability, were organised by filing and indexing the material. The analysis included the search for themes or recurring regularities, items and patterns. This involved not only the discovery of commonalities across subjects, but also a search for natural variation in the data using, for example, flow charts. The understanding that the thematic exploration provided was validated through briefing sessions involving key participants like the research assistants, and the tabulation of the frequencies with which certain themes, relations or insights were supported by the data. Also, the researchers tried to interrelate the various themes in a manner that provided an overall structure to the entire body of the data.

Documents were subjected to an analytical reading, for example, analyses of political priority and legal basis of immunization programmes, content analyses, some of them quantitative- for example, to assess the degree of bias in immunization coverage from relevant reports and quantitative analysis, for instance, tables of numbers and ledgers that provide various measures of the content, characteristics and requirements of the immunization programme and were used as a source of data on immunization services.

The researcher shifted and decoded the data from observational studies to make sense of the situation, events and interactions observed. As the data were systematically recorded, so they were also systematically analysed.

The framework for data analysis (Kaddar et al 2000) described above was used to analyse costs and financing data. In addition, in the SWOT analysis framework (SWOT stands for strengths, weaknesses, opportunities, and threats). This analysis can be used to study the strengths and weaknesses of immunisation services and the health system at each level. Also, it can be used to identify opportunities and threats from outside immunisation services and the health system that may have an effect on them) was used to complement Kadder et al's analysis framework where such a framework is deficient, such as the issues of control of financing and commitment of financing.

The analysis of the stakeholder data focused on comparing information and developing conclusions about the stakeholders' characteristics. For the resource map, the analysis involved a comparison of the factors of power, relationships, processes and accountability to provide an understanding on how the political process affects the flow and use of resources and the financial sustainability of the EPI.

Developing the resource map questionnaire

Steps similar to the ones used in developing the Stakeholder Analysis questionnaire were followed to develop the Resource Map questionnaire. First, on the basis of the traditional National Health Accounts methodology described by Rannan-Eliza et al (1997), the researcher made inventories of public and private sector organisations and agencies involved in EPI-related activities and potential information sources, as outlined above.

The list of information sources consisted of three public health inspectors providing immunization, the manager of the CISP-Italian Fund, an NGO supporting the EPI, and the officer in charge of a divisional health team. Like the stakeholder analysis tool, the process of developing the list of information sources involved consultations with members of the research team, including the health economist at the MRC and the manager and staff of the EPI, and review of the relevant literature.

Second, following the construction of the stakeholder analysis tool, the Resource Map questionnaire was developed. It focused on the flow and uses of resources within the EPI. Most importantly, questions were designed to elicit information on the issues of power, relationships, accountability and processes in the flow and use of resources--- all of great importance when one considers the financial sustainability of the EPI. The first two of these factors are Power and Resources. The other three factors are Relationships, Process and Accountability. The Concise Oxford English Dictionary (1982) defines the term relationship as state of being related; condition or character due to being related; kinship. Process is defined as a course or state of going-on, a series of events or actions, a method of operation, forward movement, to handle something following set procedures. And accountability is defined as liable, responsible, legally bound or responsible (having control over, accountable for), capable of rational conduct, trustworthy, involving responsibility. These factors can be influenced by the political strategies adopted by health reformers. A central purpose of the tool is to provide understanding on how the political process affects the flow and use of EPI resources and the financial sustainability of the EPI. Here again, the process of developing the resource map tool involved consultations with members of the research team including the health economist at the MRC and the manager and staff of the EPI, and review of the relevant literature.

Third, a pre-test of the tool was conducted with a similar focus for pretesting the Stakeholder Analysis questionnaire, and using the same interview protocol and procedures for data collection and analysis. Analysis of the resource map data involved comparing information and developing conclusions about the factors of Power and Resources, Relationships, Process and Accountability outlined above and making conclusions on how these factors affected the flow and use of EPI resources and what political strategies could be implemented to address the issues of resource flow and use.

Finally, four matrices were created to organise and present the data, as described above.

Summary

This chapter on the development and application of the resource map tool has described a similar approach to developing and applying the stakeholder analysis tool. Both of these tools and the concepts and frameworks on which they are based are, as we have seen, important elements of the SIA framework and the case study methodological which illustrates the SIA framework's role in public health policy change, the subject of this book. The following and final chapter makes some important conclusions, including a review of the contributions the book has made, and presents a discussion that includes suggestions for future work.

11

Conclusions

While there have been remarkable achievements in the EPI of particularly developing countries since 1974, attaining equitable and enduring vaccination for all children globally has not been possible. As we have seen, the international health community, and national governments to a lesser extent, has been effective in reducing the main threats of communicable diseases, however sustainability is still a major problem facing governmental as well as and non-governmental organisations health programs. Although National leaders are well aware of the limitations of child health programs, they often fail to consciously plan for sustainability (Sarriot et al 2004). This is partly because of lack of a conceptual clarity and methodological difficulties (e.g, Christopher et al 2013). However, in the past decade there had been efforts (e.g. Bossert 1990) to shed light on the conceptual confusion, making it possible for researchers to suggest practical steps that can tackle the methodological problems to assessing the sustainability of public health programmes. Despite the methodological challenges, there is great need to emphasise sustainability assessment of public health programmes because of its importance for child health and wellness (Sarriot et al 2004). The methodological approach proposed in this book can be a useful approach to measuring and improving how we deal with issues of sustainability through our immunisation programmes. This chapter elaborates these conclusions. It begins with a review of the book's contributions, then the application scenario and, finally, a discussion and future work

6.1 Review of Contributions

This book has dealt with one of the most important current challenges and complex issues of policy-based management of EPI programmes- a policy to introduce new vaccines. The following section presents the book's contributions in this respect.

Sustainability Impact Assessment

The aim of this book is to present a methodological approach for assessing the sustainability of immunization programmes that illustrates the role Sustainability Impact Assessment can play in assessment of public health policy change processes based on a case study. This role is demonstrated by the theoretical contribution Sustainability Impact Assessment makes to the methodological approach. Like the SIA, the methodological approach serves as an instrument for assessing the sustainability of proposed policies. Also, like the SIA the methodological approach and the case study on which it is based takes full account of the three sustainable development dimensions: economic, social and environmental effects of policies, strategies, plans and programmes and provides the means that all three sustainable development aspects are fully integrated into the assessment. Similar to the SIA approach, the methods of the methodological approach focus on both monetary and non-monetary approaches, and establish the procedures for conducting sustainability assessments, the decisions to be made, the methods tools and indicators to be used, who is involved and what are their responsibilities in the assessment, and the ways in which the results are disseminated. Consistent with the SIA's principle of participation, the methodological approach emphasises the involvement of stakeholders in the assessment, and the procedures for doing this. Likewise, the methodological approach seeks to create policies that consider, among other things, the political and sectoral context of the policy proposal, as well as the issues of transparency and accountability at different levels. The book's contributions are further shown by the application of the methodological approach to the particular immunisation policy change in the Gambia outlined in the foregoing discussion

Methodological Approach

Based on the premise that the sustainability of complex EPI programmes depends on many technical and organisational issues that need to be properly addressed by a sustainability policy, inspired by the sustainability impact assessment approach the book has proposed a methodological approach to support the policy process on introduction of new vaccines. As suggested by the SIA approach (EC 2003), the methodological approach focused on causal chain analysis with the aims at identifying the significant cause–effect links between the proposed introduction of new vaccines in the EPI and its eventual economic, social and environmental impacts. As we have seen, the review of literature in this study on which the methodological approach is based has demonstrated that there were no appropriate tools for the goals, objectives and questions of the study. Therefore, as mentioned, a Stakeholder Analysis questionnaire (Schmeer 1999) has been adoption, incorporating selected indicators of financial sustainability in the literature, in addition to country-specific indicators. In addition, a Resource Map Questionnaire has been developed, based on the national health accounts methodology, to complement the stakeholder analysis tool. As mentioned, use of these methodological approaches included utilisation of data from EPI, Government and donor records, and several interview and questionnaire data collection approaches. The development and use of these tools make the study most likely to, among other things; appropriately inform health policy-makers and managers of the EPI and the process of developing financial sustainability plans. This approach is consistent with the SIA methodology which suggests that there is no "one-size-fits-all" approach to sustainability impact assessment, arguing for the use of various quantitative and qualitative assessment tools (EC 2003).

In terms of contribution to international health research the methodological approach provides methods that, to the best of the writer's knowledge, have not been or are seldom used systematically before in the health field to assess the sustainability of immunization systems with regard to the issue on introduction of new vaccines the study focused on and the efficiency of having multiple organisations running programmes. Many writers (e.g., Scherer et al (2011); Christopher et al 2013) confirm this suggestion. For example, Scherer et al (2011, 12) state that:

> "research on health-related interventions has traditionally focused on the causal efficacy of the intervention itself, especially by using randomized controlled trial designs. Although evaluation literature has expanded the repertoire of methods for efficacy research to encompass several types of nonexperimental designs, the emphasis is still on the outcomes of the intervention itself, rather than on variables affecting the organizational contexts surrounding implementation and sustainability".

The use of such variables in the study focusing on the efficiency and sustainability of the EPI is important considering that the methods were used in one of the developing countries where such studies are limited. As indicated, the literature review revealed that not only was stakeholder analysis developed within generic strategic management literature and was used in the private sector to include all the groups who have an interest in the business (Winstanley et al, 1997), but it also appears that there was little use of the approach in health care in general and none in the EPI in particular. More importantly the study has provided additional methodological data to the stakeholder analysis and resource map frameworks that was not identified in the literature, such as the inclusion of indicators of financial sustainability in the stakeholder analysis and the organisation and compilation of data on questions of power, relationships, processes and accountability in the EPI in the resource map strategy.

The methodological approach will help planners of immunisation programmes in other countries identifying and managing stakeholders as described in the foregoing discussion. Also, the methodological approach provides EPI planners and policy-makers, a practical and useful approach for understanding many immunisation financing issues, such as estimating the current level of total financing for the EPI and the prospects for increasing funding; estimating the allocation of spending to priority EPI programmes and population groups; and assessing the financial importance of key players in the EPI as a guide to the development of reform strategies.

At the Gambian level, the study is most likely to appropriately inform health policy-makers and managers of the EPI and the process of developing financial sustainability plans than the usual expenditure reviews. Also, the study can provide a useful platform for staff of the Planning Unit, DOSH&SW, who were at the time considering how to use the National Health Accounts (NHA) methodology to review health expenditures in the Gambia.

Application Scenarios

As mentioned, the case study on which the methodological approach is based has assessed the sustainability of the expansion of the Expanded programme on innunisation in the Gambia, and explored whether to use additional resources for improving efficiency in the supply chain rather than introducing new vaccines which has been the government policy. In doing so the study has considered many of the requirements, actors, phases and processes involved in such a difficult process. These are some conclusions that emerged from this general accomplishment.

The application of the methodological approach in the Gambia entailed much work load as the application process included design of the tools. An important step was the definition of the objectives of the study as it has an impact on the design of the assessment. The objectives necessitated the development of the tools of the methodological approach: a stakeholder analysis questionnaire (incorporating key indicators of financial sustainability that focus both on reliable and sufficient funding for the EPI and improvement in the supply chain) and a resource map tool. Related to this step is the fact that the methodological approach provides policy-makers a systematic approach for assessing the sustainability of introducing new vaccines. For the stakeholder analysis the researcher systematically gathered and analysed qualitative information to determine whose interests should be taken into account, but more importantly to assess where people think the system works and where it doesn't work, and if different parties have contradictory incentives. This way the researcher was able to analyse stakeholder characteristics on the issue of whether to use the limited resources to introduce new vaccines, or use such resources to improve the weak EPI infrastructure, as described especially in Chapter 9. Using the resource map framework the researcher described in detail the flow of resources and expenditures and how they are used within the immunisation system, as also described in Chapter 10. As indicated, the researcher used the strategy of resource mapping to organise and compile data that focus on questions of power, relationships, processes and accountability in the EPI. This approach is generally lacking in assessments of health care strategies, expenditures and policies. Also, as indicated the use of data from the EPI, Government and donor records, and several interview and questionnaire data collection approaches added to this integrated approach that helped the researcher collect data from various sources needing various approaches, as outlined above.

As mentioned, the research was conducted in the context of change in the health system in general and the EPI in particular. It coincided with the development of a financial sustainability plan for the EPI, the first of its kind in the country. As such, the study was an opportunity to let stakeholders discuss and assess their experiences and to reflect on what should be done now and in the future. Thus, the timeline for assessment of sustainability was in line with the needs of decision-makers, which is an important requirement for such assessment (OECD, 2010; Langer et al 2002)

Strength of the study with respect to applying the methodological approach is the pre-testing and development and using the tools. As already indicated, the methodology of developing and using the tools consisted of several steps of identifying information sources, conducting interviews and creating tools from generic frameworks. These steps culminated in a period of piloting and refining of the methodology and the tools. As mentioned above, this exercise produced methods that had seldom been used systematically before to assess the sustainability of systems immunisation programmes, and can better inform immunisation policy change processes. The need for such an approach is highlighted by the literature which shows not only the lack of tools for measuring the sustainability of public health programmes but also systematic approaches to tool development. For example, in their literature review of 85 relevant studies focusing on program sustainability in public health, Schell et al (2013) identified only two out of 53 peer-reviewed articles that developed a tool to assess program sustainability. Of the tools that do exist, none have been successfully tested for reliability or validity, nor have the developed measures been retested in subsequent studies.

Discussion & Future work

We have presented a methodological approach for assessing the sustainability of the expansion of the EPI to illustrate the role sustainability impact assessment can play in community health policy change and demonstrated its application to the EPI progrmmme in the Gambian. This section further discusses several factors that are relevant for the suggestion of this novel methodological approach to assessing sustainability in relation to the intricate issue of immunization which is an important aspect of child health in particularly developing countries. Concerning the Sustainability Impact Assessment methodology that contributes the main theoretical framework to the methodological approach, and the Stakeholder analysis and Resource map frameworks that the SIA methodology includes, a number of issues deserve additional discussion.

As we have seen, the tools of the SIA and methodological approaches are not only instruments for assessing the sustainability of proposed policies, they also considers the three sustainable development dimensions of economic, social and environmental sustainability and their influence on policies, etc, and provides ways all these three sustainability aspects are combined in the assessment. The relevance of this approach to assessing sustainability in public health has been widely articulated in the relevant literature. For example, Sarriot et al (2004p14) argue that "we need to place sustainability evaluation at the center of child health programmes, not because of fads or inclination for development buzzwords, but simply because we measure what we value and often value what we measure. If we are serious about child hood survival and –ultimately-child health and wellbeing….we need to value, measure and improve how we deal with sustainability through our health programmes". Also, Christopher et al (2013, p10) suggest that for the idea [of sustainability]to have meaning, it is important that it be more sharply delimited by concentrating it on population health which, as we have seen in Chapter 1, is closely related to public health. Another way this can be done is through including other evaluative criteria that should inform healthcare policy and planning, such as effectiveness, efficacy, responsiveness, and equity. On the importance of including the three pillars of sustainability in sustainability assessment of public health policy development the methodological approach, as we have seen, has focused on three current social, financing and environmental sustainability debates/issues and how they relate to the case study (Chapters 7-10) as outlined in chapter 1, as examples of issues that can precede sustainability related to public health. These social, economic and environmental issues, as mentioned, are ethics, the global marketplace and healthcare financing, including the issues of structural adjustments and governance as they relate to sustainability in health care in general and the EPI in particular. The methodological approach is a step in these directions. The institutional and methodological difficulties that including these three pillars of sustainable development pose should be tackled, as already mentioned, through trying and learning to improve methodologies, as suggested by the SIA methodology (EC 2003)

Using the methodological approach proposed here countries can address the issue of whether to use limited resources for introducing new vaccines or rather to use the limited resources to improve EPI infrastructure, or to do so after improving the EPI infrastructure. This approach no doubt helps in providing policy-makers as well as other stakeholders information needed in making such a decision in especially resource-constrained environments, where sustainability of the EPI matter most.

There are many lessons from the case study for public health professionals who want to influence the policy change process. The case study showed that knowledge about a policy issue can influence the policy process, as Buse et al (2005, p111) explains:

> "Within a policy sub-system or community, two sets of motivation guide the actions of groups involved in policy formulation: knowledge or expertise and material interest (Howlett and Ramesh 2003). Thus membership of a discourse community (sometimes known as an 'epistemic community') is defined by shared political values and a shared understanding of a problem, its definition and its causes, though usually marked by detailed disagreements about policy responses, whereas an interest network is based on some common material interest.... Both discourse communities and interest networks operate in the health policy sub-system since both ideas and interests play a part in policy change. When discourse and interest networks are closely linked, stable and cohesive, the policy sub-system will be less amenable to new policy options. Shared understandings of the nature of the policy problem and the range of feasible responses are difficult to change once established"

The majority of stakeholders in the study who, as shown by the responses of the stakeholders, are generally knowledgeable about the issue of whether to introduce new vaccines or instead use the limited resources to improve the EPI infrastructure and funding, strongly support the latter option and, therefore, the sustainability of the EPI, because they feel that adding new vaccines to the weak EPI would mean, among other things, additional costs that could affect the efficiency and sustainability of the EPI.

The above explanation (Buse et al 2005) also relates to another lesson to be learned. This is that ideology can influence the stance stakeholder or actors take in the political process, as identified by other writers, for example, Bryant (2002) who suggests that such findings have serious implications for all policy fields. The case study showed that the ideology of actors in the immunisation system trying to bring about a specific kind of policy change can influence their access to the political process and the receptivity of the government by their experiences and the evidence they can bring to bear on the policy change process. By using their experiences and evidence of providing immunisation services often under difficult conditions with limited resources, the immunisation providers in the case study sought to be representative of larger groups of public health workers trying to effect responsive policy change. Generally, providers are faced with several problems that affect their effectiveness and, therefore, the efficiency of the EPI and providers have many proposals to the problems that they consider the best use of additional resources, such as improvement of the cold chain system.

Another related lesson to be learned is that though stakeholders' official positions can influence how they view a policy issue, but this may not necessarily exclude other considerations. Depending on the position they occupy in Governmental and non-governmental organisations, such as UNICEF, stakeholders in the case study support or oppose the issue of whether to use limited resources for improving the weak EPI infrastructure not for introducing new vaccines. However, the majority of stakeholders want to see the EPI's infrastructure improved, irrespective of the positions they hold in their organisations, and they would also press for such improvement before any attempt to introduce new vaccines.

Another lesson to be learned is how politics can operate on the policy process. Stakeholders' interests, alliances, resources and leadership, usually related to their positions, can influence the policy process on an issue. In the case study stakeholders' interests, alliances, resources and leadership reflect their positions on the issue, with stakeholders funding new vaccines and pressuring for their introduction, such as the Global Alliance for Vaccines and Immunisation (GAVI), as well as those in Government at policy levels tending to oppose the idea of using the limited resources to improve the infrastructure first, because this excludes introduction of new vaccines, while service providers tend to place more emphasis on the need to improve the EPI infrastructure and funding. Buse et al (2005, p20) explains such a situation:

> "Resistance is not surprising if you think of policy making as a struggle between groups with competing interests, some in favour of change and others opposed to it, depending on their interests or ideas. For example, health economists often wish to limit the professional autonomy of the medical profession so as to control spending patterns. Yet such reforms are often opposed by doctors – some of whom are concerned that this will usurp their professional authority and others because it may affect their income. Policy making is, therefore, often characterized by conflicts that arise when change is proposed or pursued which threatens the status quo. The outcome of any conflict depends on the balance of power between the individuals and groups involved and the processes or rules established to resolve those conflicts".

This explanation also applies to another lesson to be learned on how both power and politics based on resource provision can influence the policy process. During the period 1997 to 2003 yearly contribution of each of the actors in the Gambian EPI has been irregular, and generally the contribution of donors remained greater than that of Government throughout the period. While the proportion of donor financing increased considerably, due primarily to spending on vaccines by GAVI, the proportion of Government's financing decreased greatly, due to poor economic climate. Despite stakeholders' interests, generally there appears to be a clear recognition of the important role donors play, so both supporters and opponents of the issue would ally with organisations providing funding for the EPI, including donors like GAVI that pressures for the introduction of new vaccines. Bruce et al (2005, p148) provides an explanation:

> "The growth of global civil society has been embraced for a number of reasons. For some it is welcomed due to the declining capacity of some states to manage policy domains – such as health. For others, it is a means to improve the policy process – by bringing new ideas and expertise into the process, by reducing conflict, improving communication or transparency. For others, civil society involvement provides the means to democratize the international system – to give voice to those affected by policy decisions thereby making these policies more responsive. Civil society is also thought to engage people as global citizens and to 'globalize from below'. Others equate civil society as pursuing humane forms of governance; providing a counterweight to the influence of the commercial sector. Despite these promises, there are others who are less sanguine".

Related to this is how resources are distributed within the immunization system, which also concern issues of management, equity and accountability. Resources pass through one main intermediary, the Ministry of Health & SW (MOH&SW), which in turn transfers resources on to the ultimate providers of services. There was increased spending in health facilities, which is consistent with service delivery in such facilities, but there was a relatively higher weight of spending in public facilities when compared to spending in private facilities. Most of the expenditure is utilized in facilities for the activity of vaccine supply and quality (mainly for the introduction of new vaccines that is supported by GAVI), with private facilities receiving a relatively smaller share of the expenditure. There were little or no expenditures on activities that enhance programme efficiency, such as research and evaluation, and monitoring and supervision activities in both public and private facilities, and none on programme management in private facilities.

Another related issue that provides another lesson to be learned is the nature of decision-making in the immunisation system. As mentioned, decision-making on EPI expenditure varies according to the level at which decisions are made, with officials of donors and Government making decisions on the use of EPI resources based on Government policy, prepared projects and budgets (usually without the involvement of providers at the periphery of health care), and donor conditions, while the use of EPI funds at the provider level, particularly at the level of the health facility, are predetermined by decisions taken at central level.

Buse et al (2005) suggest that power as decision making concentrates on actions of individuals and groups which operate on policy decisions. Buse et al (2005) cite Robert Dahl's classic study, Who Governs?, which concentrated on the issue of who made important decisions on contested issues in New Haven, Connecticut, USA (Dahl 1961, cited by Buse et al 2005). Through analysing the preferences of interest groups and comparing them with policy impacts, Dahl drew conclusions about who had power. Dahl was able to find that there were various resources which gave power to interest groups and citizens, and that such resources were distributed unevenly. Individuals, who had much political resources, possessed less of the other resources. This made it possible for various individuals and groups to influence dissimilar policy issues. Dahl's (as cited Buse et al 2005, p 21) conclusion from these findings is that "different groups in society, including weak groups, could 'penetrate' the political system and exercise power over decision makers in accordance with their preferences. While only a few people had direct influence over key decisions, defined as successfully initiating or vetoing policy proposals, most had indirect influence by the power of the vote".

According to Buse et al (2005), Dahl used a long list of potential assets to define the meaning of political resources. Dahl identified access to cash, social standing, legal trappings linked to holding official office, credit and wealth, control over information and jobs as especially significant in this policy environment. As Buse et al (2005) suggest, there are various resources that actors can use in health policy that will be an action of the specific policy environment and content.

Therefore, creating collective agreement and opinion reached by stakeholders in the immunization system is important (consensus building) for action; initiating action on decisions taken necessitates the overall understanding of the causes and effects (awareness building), and the active involvement of all relevant stakeholders to discuss and debate the issues concerned (review and hearings). Such decision-making also includes issues like ownership, visioning, flexibility, empowerment, informed consent, community choice etc. Such approaches, as we have seen, are consistent with the principles of sustainability in public health. As the WHO (WHO 1998) indicates, public health activities should:

- enable individuals and communities to gain more power over the personal, socioeconomic and environmental factors that affect their health;
- involve those who are concerned about an issue in all stages of project planning, implementation and evaluation; and
- be guided by a concern for equity and social justice.

To achieve such goals there is need for consensus building, awareness building, and review and hearings. Immunisation policy decisions that are made by governments, stakeholders and communities are more likely to have broad and lasting impact.

One factor favoring both the sustainability impact assessment approach and the methodological approach's acceptability is that they, as we have seen in previous chapters, include methods and tools that are individually now being well promoted by international agencies, governments and the health research community. Also, the approaches are non-prescriptive about the tools and methods that need to be used in the measurement of the elements in the different sustainability dimensions. The premise on which the methodological approach is based concurs with writers (eg, Scheirer 2011) who suggest that sustainability of health projects cannot be looked at within a purely biological view, but rather in a much broader perspective of human, social and organizational processes. It is necessary to deal with the non-linerality and complexity of health programme environments (The most central start point for complexity is that it is about non-linearity. That means prediction and control is often not possible, perhaps harmful, or at least not useful as ideas for understanding programmes operating in complex environments (Censemaking 2014). In

Chapter 2 we have outlined different views about what sustainability is and what can be done to advance it, and suggested that in spite of all the controversy there seem to be three interrelated categories of sustainability that are used to examine global issues which this book adapts: social sustainability, economic and financial sustainability and environmental sustainability. We have also seen that the conceptual framework on which this methodological approach is based shows that the issue of sustainability of the EPI cannot be divorced from the political and economic climate surrounding a health programme, both in the local context, and in the wider national and international context. Some of the most common threats to the sustainability of the EPI in relation to the government, for example, are government bureaucratic procedures, currency devaluation, unfavourable political climate and long-term global trends. These proposals correspond with the suggestion that most planning models that are linear in the conventional input-process-output –outcome form does not interpret the non-linear reality of how sustainability exists in areas such as public health within which the case study was implemented. Factors that enhance sustainability in this view that have been widely included in multidimensional frameworks for planning and evaluation are urging performance to build capacity, achieved or perceived health progress that can affect the adoption of new behaviors, as well as cause and effect in relationships, such as social capital, trust and the willingness to collaborate at the community or inter-organizational levels. The methodological approach integrates a wider perspective of sustainability to assess the sustainability of EPI systems and the efficiency of having multiple organisations running programmes which makes it more meaningful to the process of sustainability planning and evaluation in the EPI.

Among the drawbacks of the methodological approach is the "neutrality" of the researcher and the truth of responses (Richardson, 1997) that are associated with the qualitative approach is a weakness. The stakeholder analysis framework is not focused on statistical generalisations; rather it aims at reflecting the perceptions and feelings of those interviewed. In this application, respondents represented the views of various types of stakeholders within and outside the health sector in the Gambia. We have also seen in chapter 5 that the NHA framework on which the resource map strategy is based is not the answer to all health policy questions. One limitation of NHAs is that health accounts do not distinguish between effective and ineffective expenditures. Therefore, to answer many policy questions, NHA information must be combined with non-financial data, such as those suggested by the SIA approach (Chapter 6).

This is the approach followed in the case study through combining the resource map strategy with a stakeholder analysis framework that includes indicators to assess the sustainability of the policy issue in the immunization system. This methodological approach looks at the sustainability of immunisation service delivery organizations including their effectiveness, efficacy, responsiveness and equity, as well as capturing several processes that may be relevant to the development of sustainable immunization programmes. Also, it incorporates models based on financial self-reliance which are valuable at the organizational, as well as other models that are in touch with the global context (e.g., external sources of financing) in which programmes operate. Some stakeholders in the case study indicated that "users" as important stakeholders should have been included in the study. The addition of indirect costs borne by mothers who take their children to clinics for immunizations and their opinions about the service, for example, would have provided a better understanding of the flow of uses of resources within the immunization system and other issues that influence their use of the service. As required in such impact assessments, the researcher should ensure that the principle of stakeholder involvement and consultation is applied more widely and effectively (Abaza 2003). However, the involvement and participation of stakeholders in the study was limited to priority stakeholders at the central, secondary and primary levels of health care. This was because the focus of the study was mainly on the supply side of the immunisation services, not on the demand side which would have required the involvement of other kinds of stakeholders. Furthermore, though involvement of a wide range of actors from government and civil society can provide data, insights and information that is not available to policy analysts working in isolation, there are, however, a number of difficulties and constraints that can occur when promoting stakeholder participation that were considered in the case study, such as identification and inclusion of all interested and affected parties, and time/cost implications of dealing with such problems (Abaza 2003).

Toman et al (1998) also point to two somewhat related conceptual and practical challenges in assessing sustainability that must be taken into account (Chapter 2&6). One is the problem of determining which physical scales to use for sustainability assessments when there are multiple and overlapping communities or stakeholder groups. Another is the criteria to be used, in particular the relationship between sustainability and measures of economic wellbeing and the use of monetary versus nonmonetary indicators. The case study demonstrates not only these challenges but also the possibilities of overcoming them through, for example, developing multi-criteria strategies and processes of stakeholder involvement. Future work could be directed to better understanding of these problems, especially how to assess sustainability in practice at multiple scales which Toman et al suggest remains less well understood. For example, future users of the methodological approach should consider in planning such assessments including some kind of wider community participation and stakeholder involvement in the assessment with a view to gaining better insight into these challenges.

Cost data used in this application scenario were based on the assumptions described in the national Financial Sustainability Plan (FSP) (2003) of the country. These and other estimates obtained at the central level might have been exaggerated or under-estimated. Similarly, some cost data obtained from the divisional and facility levels of the system, particularly the facility level, might have been insufficient due to factors like poor record keeping. These are also drawbacks that future users of the methodological approach should consider.

Of particular importance is dealing with the politics and ethics of policy analysis. The policy analysis tools used in the case study demand creativity and evidence as well as judgement. Also, the tools are filled with ethical questions and values (Bruce et al 2005). Political and ethical difficulties for policy analysis are outlined by Bruce et al (2005, p189-190):

> "...Policy change is political and ...analysis for policy typically serves political ends. Making policy alternatives and their consequences more explicit and improving the political feasibility of policy are neither value-neutral nor immune to politics. Policy analysis, therefore, will not invariably lead to better policy (e.g. policy which improves efficiency, equity or addresses problems of public health importance), or to better policy processes (e.g. fair decision making processes in which all stakeholders are provided opportunities to air their views and influence decisions). The substance and process of policy analysis are influenced by who finance, executes and interprets the analysis... Analysis of a policy can be a resource intensive endeavour. Not all policy actors are endowed with resources. Everything else being equal, policy analysis may serve to reinforce the prevailing distribution of power and economic resources: those with political resources are more likely to be those who can finance analysis and influence who will use the analysis and how it will be used. Those groups with more political resources are in a better position to develop political strategies to manage the positions, players, power and perceptions surrounding a policy issue. In this way, policy analysis may reinforce the status quo.
>
> Policy analysis is influenced not just by interests and power but also by interpretation. These issues raise questions about the role of the analyst, or of the organization for which the analyst works, in the analysis. If the analysis is for policy, it is almost inevitable that the analyst will have a

preferred policy outcome. The policy goal may be at odds with 'good policy' as discussed above (e.g. many well-intentioned health professionals champion causes with poor cost-effectiveness). As no-one is value neutral; it is difficult to produce policy analysis which is unbiased. While there are ways to minimize bias, for example, by triangulating methods and sources of information and testing results with peers, it is probably necessary to accept the fact that the results of policy analysis will be biased.

Policy analysis raises other kinds of ethical issues. For example, is it ethical to allow any group to participate in the policy process so as to develop a more powerful coalition? Is it ethical to undermine the legitimacy of opponents or to withhold information from public discourse for tactical purposes? How far should one compromise on policy preferences so as to accommodate and win over a policy opponent? Your values will dictate how you answer these questions. In thinking about your response it may be useful to assume that other actors use these and other techniques to manipulate the substance and process of policy to their advantage. This may lead you to decide to join in the process of strategically managing the policy process to achieve your aims. Alternatively, you may feel uncomfortable with some of the strategies and decide that the ends do not justify the means. While these means may relate to values and ethics, they may also relate to the time, resources and emotional costs of pursuing, and at times failing to achieve, a particular policy change. There is nothing inherently wrong with abandoning or adopting a political strategy – particularly as it will now be based on a solid grasp of the fact that successful policy change requires a political approach".

To tackle such methodological and other difficulties the sustainability Impact Assessment approach guidelines emphasise the need for researchers to engage in learning- by- doing to improve methodologies (EU 2003). There is considerable potential for deliberation, social learning and innovation from a more open and pluralistic assessment process. This leads to better practice and more sound integrated policies, thereby enhancing sustainable development. This is a recurring theme in chapters of this book where such methodological problems are discussed. As we have seen, the SIA approach itself tries to deal with these methodological issues in several ways. For example, it considers the need for establishing clear procedures on who is responsible for which steps in the SIA and the decision-making process, what methods, tools and indicators will be used, which stakeholders and experts have to be involved and in what way, and how the results will be presented and to whom. However, as Bruce et al (2005, 190) conclude "While analysis may more often serve to reinforce the status quo, without the use of policy analysis tools groups without power will remain at a perpetual disadvantage".

While the case study methodological approach gives promising guidelines for measuring complex processes such as organisational capacity and leadership, indicators focusing on larger environmental and social issues have been less covered. These measurement areas which demand large quantities of qualitative work can usefully be incorporated in future assessment efforts that must concentrate on developing the needed measurement tools which are currently lacking in the health field (Lafond et al 2002). The methodological approach could be revised to address these challenging issues that will enable its policy assessment process to focus more on contextual information from particularly the community to influence the policy process. This requires consideration of the SIA principles and guidelines, including the practical points for the implementation of the SIA approach outlined in Chapter six.

As we have seen, sustainability is a major challenge for both governments and NGOs partly because of lack of clarity of its meaning and the methodological problems linked to the assessment of sustainability. However, we have also seen that there have been efforts in the last three decades to resolve, for instance, the conceptual difficulties associated with sustainability that can lead to practical steps to deal with the methodological problems. A general conclusion and future work of this book is that much more effort is required to assess the sustainability of immunization systems. The SIA and case study methodological approaches, like most disciplines of social science, seek to provide approaches to better comprehend a very complex and unpredictable health environment. Experience in assessing and sustaining capacity development for health outcomes is still limited (Hacker 2012). Inspired by the SIA approach this methodological approach provides one way to help categorise information into broad dimensions and components in order to help public health practitioners and policy-makers better understand the variables and determinants that will influence the sustainability of their actions.

Bibliography

Abaza, H (2003). The role of integrated assessment in achieving sustainable development. Geneva: Economics and Trade Branch, UN Environment Programme.

Academy of Finland .(2003). Nursing and caring sciences evaluation report. Available at http://www.aka.fi/globalassets/awanhat/documents/tiedostot/julkaisut/12_03-hoitotieteen-arviointi.pdf

Africa Development Bank .(2016). Gambia Economic Outlook. Available at: https://www.afdb.org › Home › Countries › West Africa › Gambia

Akumu AO, English M, Scott JA, Griffiths UK . (2007). Economic evaluation of delivering Haemophilus influenzae type b vaccine in routine immunization services in Kenya. Bull of the World Health Organisation. 07 July; 85(7):511-8.;

Albright, M.K. (1997). State Department first annual report on environmental diplomacy in entering the century of the environment:A new social contract for science. Science 279: 491-497

Association of Faculties of Medicine of Canada. (1995). Part 1 - Theory: thinking about health. Chapter 4: Basic Concepts in Prevention, Surveillance, and Health. Available at http://phprimer.afmc.ca/Part1-TheoryThinkingAboutHealth/Chapter4BasicConceptsInPreventionSurveillanceAndHealthPromotion/Thestagesofprevention

Altman, D.G. Sustaining interventions in community systems: on the relationship between researchers and communities. Health Psychol. 1995;14(6):526–5. Available at http://www.aka.fi/Tiedostot/Tiedostot/Jul kaisut/12_03%20Hoitotieteen%20arviointi.pdf

Batson, A. (1998). Sustainable introduction of affordable new vaccines: the targeting strategy. Washington D. C, USA: World Bank

Berger, G. (2007). Sustainability impact assessment: approaches and applications in Europe. ESDN, Quarterly Reports, the European Sustainable Development Network. Available at www.sd-network.eu › Quarterly reports

Blair J.D, Rock TT, Rotarius TM, Fottler MD, Bosse GC, Driskill JM. (1996a). The problematic fit of diagnosis and strategy for medical group stakeholders – including IDS/Ns. Health Care Management Review 21(1): 7–28.

Blair JD, Fottler MD, Whitehead CJ. 1996b. Diagnosing the stakeholder bottom line for medical group practices:key stakeholders'potential to threaten and/or cooperate. Medical GroupManagement Journal 43(2): 40, 42–8, 50–1.

Bhatia, M., & Rifkin, S. (2010). A renewed focus on primary health care: revatilise or reframe?. London: Department of Social Policy, London School of Hygiene and Tropical Medicine

Burton, S. (1999). Evaluation of healthy city projects: stakeholder analysis of two projects in
Bangladesh. Environment and Urbanization, 11(1), 41-52.

BikiCrumba. (2006). Characteristics of the new public health approach. Available at www. boredofstudies.org/wiki/characteristics-of-the-new-public--A

Boundris, A.(2015). Improving health through primary health care and public health collaboration. McMaster, Canada: McMaster University school of Nursing. Available at www.nursing.mcmaster.ca/news.story 105.html

Blasinsky, M;, Goldman H.H; and Unutzer J. Project impact: a report on barriers and facilitators to sustainability. Adm. Policy Ment. Health. 2006;33 (6):718–729.

Brughla, R and Varvasovszky, Z. (2000). Stakeholder analysis: a review. Health Policy and Planning;15 (3): 239–246

Bryant, T .(1986). Role of knowledge in public health and health promotion policy change. Health Promot. Int. (2002) 17 (1): 89-98. doi: 10.1093/ heapro/17.1.89

Brownson, R. C;. Chriqui, J.F and Stamatakis, K.A. (2009). Understanding evidence-based public health policy. Am J Public Health. 2009 September; 99 (9): 1576–1583. doi: 10.2105/AJPH.2008.156224

Bossert, T.J. (1990). Can they get along without us?: sustainability of donor-supported health projects in Central America and Africa. Soc Sci Med. 1990;30(9):1015-23.

Buse, k; Mays, N and Walt, G. (2005). Making health policy. Open University Press

Canadian Public Health Association. (1996). Action Statement for Health Promotion in Canada. Montroel :CPHA. Available at http://www.cpha.ca/en/ programs/policy/action.aspx

Cassels A (1997). A guide to sector-wide approaches for health development: concepts, issues and working arrangements. WHO, Danida: Dfid, EC. WHO/ ARA/97.12.

Carrin, G; Buse, K and Quah, S.R. (2008). Health system policy, finance and organisation. Elsevier and Academic Press

Censemaking. (2014). Developmental Evaluation and Complexity. Available at: | https://censemaking.com/2014/01/10/developmental-evaluation-and-complexity/

Center for Disease Control and Prevention. (2015). Definition of policy, Available at www.cdc.gov/policy/analysis/process definition.html

Center for Disease Control and Prevention. (1999). Ten great public health

achievements-United States, 1900-1999 MMWR, April 02/48(12); 241-243.
Center for Disease control and Prevention. (2011). What is health marketing ?. CDC 1600 Chfton Rd, Atlanta GA 30333, USA. Available at http://www. Cdc.gov/health communication /tools tem/
Century, J., Rudnick M and Freeman, C. (2010). A framework for measuring fidelity of implementation: a foundation for shared language and accumulation of knowledge. Am J Eval. 2010;31(2):199–218
Christopher, G., Hudson, I and Yvonne, M. (2013). Sustainability at the edge of choas: its limits and possibilities in public health. Biomed Research International, Vol 2013(2013), Article ID 801614. Available at http:// dx.doi.org/10.1155/2013/801614
Christopher, H., J. L. Murray, David B. Evans. Health Systems Performance Assessment: debates, methods and empiricism. WHO/Amazon.Com
Cross, H., Hardee, K and Jewell, N. (2001). Reforming operational policies: a pathway to improving reproductive health Programmes." Policy Occasional Paper #7.Washington, DC: Futures Group, Policy Project.
Cutts, F.T., Zaman, S.M,, Enwere ,G., Jaffar, S., Levine, O.S., Okoko, J.B., Oluwalana, C., Vaughan, A., Obaro, S.K., Leach, A., McAdam, K.P., Biney, E., Saaka, M., Onwuchekwa, U., Yallop, F., Pierce, N.F., Greenwood, B.M and Adegbola, RA. (2005). Efficacy of nine-valent pneumococcal conjugate vaccine against pneumonia and invasive pneumococcal disease in The Gambia: randomised, double-blind, placebo-controlled trial. Lancet. 2005 Mar 26-Apr 1;365(9465):1139-46.
Columbia University. (2005). An expanded definition of sustainability. Columbia, USA: Columbia University's Biosphere 2 center
Costello, A., Watson, F. and Woodward, D. (1994). Human face or human façade?: adjustment and the health of mothers and children. Occasional Paper, Institute of Child Health, London

Dahlgren, G and Whitehead, M. (1991) Social model of health. Available at http://www.nwci.ie/download/pdf/determinants_health_diagram.pdf
Department of Immunization, Vaccines and Biologicals. (2002). The common assessment tool for immunization services.Geneva : World Health Organization. Available at http://www.who.int/iris/handle/10665/68871
Dearing, J.W. (2009). Applying diffusion of innovation theory to intervention development. Res Soc Work Pract. 2009;19(5):503–518.]
Dearing, J.W and Kreuter, M.W. (2010). Designing for diffusion of cancer communication innovations. Patient Educ Couns. 2010;81(suppl 1):S100–S110.
Damschroder, LJ., Aron, D.C., Keith, R.E., Kirsh, S.R., Alexander, J.A and

Lowery, J.C. (2009). Fostering implementation of health services research findings into practice: a consolidated framework for advancing implementation science. Implement Sci. 2009;4:50.]

Davidson, M.L(1983). Multidimensional Scaling. New York: John WIley and Sons, Inc; 1983.

Department of Health. (2014). Primary and community health. Department of health, State Government of Victoria, Australia. Available at http://www.health.vic.gov.au/pch/

Dictionary. Com. (2017). Human Capital. Available at http://www.dictionary.com/browse/human-capital

Doherty, J. (2015). Effective capacity-building strategies for health technology assessment ... Available at: www.idsihealth.org/.../Doherty-2016-Effective-CB-for-HTA_reviewFINAL-24-2-16....

Donaldson, C & Gerard, K (1993). Economics of healthcare financing: the visible hand. London: Macmillan Press.

Edvardsson, K., Garvars, R., Ivarsson, A., Euremius, E., Mogren, I and Nystrum . M.E. (2011). Sustainable practice change; professionals experience with a multisectoral child health promotion programme in Sweden. BMC health serv.Res. 2011 Mar 22.11.61. dol: 10.1186/1472-6963-11-61

Elseman, E and Fossum, D. (2005). The challenges of creating a global health resource tracking system. Rand Corporation, Amazon.Com

Environmental Protection Agency. (2011). Sustainability and the US EPA: Chapter 4-Sustainability Assessment and Management: Process, Tools and Indicators. The National Academy of Science. Available at https://www.nap.edu/read/13152/chapter/6.

European Academy of Nursing Science. (2008). Important future topics in nursing research. Future nursing EANS report of EANS electronic survey to identify nursing/midwifery research priorities and the role of EANS. Available at available at www.european□academy□of□nursing□science.com

European Communities. (2003). Socio-economic tools for sustainability impact assessment: the contribution of EU research to sustainable development. Available at ec.europa.eu/research/social/pdf/other-pubs/socio-economic-tools-for-s.

European Union (2003). Handbook for sustainability impact assessment. Available at http://trade.ec.europa.eu/doclib/html/122363.htm

Favin, M., Macabasco, R and Steinglass, R. (2012). Impact of new vaccine introduction on developing country immunization programmes and health systems. Executive Summary for April 2012 SAGE Meeting: Grey Literature Review USAID/MCHIP (Maternal and Child Health Integrated Programme)

Bibliography

Favin M., Steinglass R., Fields R., Banerjee, K and Sawhney, M. (2012). Why children are not vaccinated: a review of the grey literature. Int. Health. 2012;4:229–238.

Fagans,P., Simmons, R & Ghiron, L. (2006). Helping public sector health system innovate: the strategic approach to strengthening reproductive health policies and programmes.AJPH 96(3): 435- 40.

Frequently asked questions from the preamble to the Constitution of the World Health Organization as adopted by the International Health Conference, 1946. Geneva: WHO

Friedman, L and Miles, S. (2006). Stakeholders theory and practice. Oxford University Press

Gambia Bureau of Statistics. (2017). 2013 Census. Kanifing: GBoS.

Global Alliance for Vaccine and Immunisation. (2000). Immunise every child: GAVI strategies for sustainable immunization services. GAVI. Available at http://www.vaccinealliance.org/resources/2nd.mtg.rept-2.pdf

George, C.(ed). (2007). Impact assessment and sustainable development: european practice and experience. Available at: http://www.e-elgar.com/shop/impact-assessment-and-sustainable-development?___website=uk_warehouse

Golladan, F.L. (1980). Community healthcare in developing countries. Finance Dev, September: 17(3):35-39

Goodman, R.M., McLeroy, K.R., Steckler, A.B and Hoyle, R.H. (1993). Development of level of institutionalization scales for health promotion programmes. Health Educ Q. 1993;20(2):161–178.

Green, L.W and Ottoson, J.M. (1999). Community and population health, 8th ed. New York and Toronto: WCB/McGraw-Hill.

Gruen, R.L, Elliott, J.H., Nolan, M.L et al. Sustainability science: an integrated approach for health-programme planning. Lancet. 2008;372(9649):1579–1589.

Goodland, R and H Daly. (1996). Environmental sustainability: universal and non-negotiable. Ecological Applications, 6: 1002-1017

Hacker, K. (2012). Community Capacity Building and Sustainability: Outcomes of ...Available at: https://www.ncbi.nlm.nih.gov/pmc/articles/PMC355784

Hall, A.J. (1990). The Gambia Hepatitis Intervention Study. MRC News, 47:36-37.

Hall, P. A., Land, H., Parker, R and Webb, A (1975). Change, choice and conflict in social policy. Lon-don: Heinemann

Hall, P. A. (1993) Policy paradigms, social learning, and the state: the case of economic policymaking in Britain..Comparative Politics 25, 275–296.

Hall, AJ, Robertson, R.L, Crivelli, P.E, Lowe, Y., Inskip, H., Snow, S.K.,Whittle, H. (1993). Cost-effectiveness of hepatitis B vaccine in The Gambia. Transactions of the Royal Society of Tropical Medicine and Hygiene 87: 333–6

Hardee, K., Ashford, L., Rottach, E., Jolivet, R and Kiesel, R. 2012. The Policy Dimensions of Scaling Up Health Initiatives. Washington, DC: Futures Group, Health Policy Project. Available at http://www.healthpolicyproject.com/pubs/83_ScaleupPolicyJuly.pdf

Henry, B.M & Cheng, W.Y. (1998). Nursing research and priorities in Africa, Asia and Europe. Journal of Nursing Scholarship 30(2):115□6

Hinman, A.R. (1999). Economic aspects of vaccines and immunizations. Les Comptes rendus de l'Académie des Sciences III322(100): 989-984, November 1999

Hyde, T.B., Dentz, H., Wang, S.A., Burchett, H.E., Mounier-Jack, S and Mantel, C.F .(2012).The impact of new vaccine introduction on immunization and health systems: a review of the published literature. Vaccine. 2012 Oct 5;30 (45):6347-58. doi: 10.1016/j.vaccine.2012.08.029. Epub 2012 Aug 29.

Inspiration Software Inc. (2015). Teaching and learning with concept maps. Available at www inspiration.com/visual learning/concept-mapping

Institute of Medicine. (1988).The future of public health. Washington, DC: National Academy Press; 1988. Available at http://www.cdc.gov/nphpsp/essentialServices.html

International Working Group for M&EED (2006): A Guide to monitoring and evaluation for energy projects. Monitoring and evaluation in energy for development. Available at http://www.gvepinternational.org/sites/default/files/resources/MEED_Guide_final_version_english.pdf

International Association of National Public Health Institutes. (2007). National public health institutes core functions. Available at www. Ianphi.org/documents/pdfs/Eire Functions IANBHI Brief.pdf#page=2&250M=a1

International Council of Nurses. (1999). Position Statement on Nursing Research. Available at http://www. icn.ch/psresearch99.htm

Irny, S.I. and Rose, A.A. (2005) "Designing a strategic information system planning methodology for malaysian institutes of higher learning (isp- ipta), Issues in Information System, Volume VI, No. 1, 2005.

Jachelson, K. (2005). From nanny to steward: the role of governance in public health. London: Kings Fund

Bibliography

Kaddar, M., Lydon, P and Levine, R.(2004). Financial challenges of immunization: a look at GAVI. Bulletin of the World Health Organization 82: 697–702

Kaddar, M., Dougherty, L., Maceira, D et al. (2000). Costs and financing of immunization programmes: findings of four case studies, Special Initiatives Report 26, Bethesda, MD: Partnerships for Health Reform Project, Abt Associates Inc.

Kates, R.W and Paris T.M. (2003). Long-term trends and sustainability transistion. New York, USA: The National Academy of Sciences, 100(14):8062-8067

Katz, E (editor). !963). The characteristics of innovations and the concept of compatibility. Paper presented at the Rehovoth Conference on Comprehensive Planning of Agriculture in Developing Countries; August 19–29, 1963; Rehovoth, Israel

Kindig, D and Stoddart, G. (2003). What is population health. Am J Public Health, March; 93(3):380-383.

Kingdon, J . W. (1984). Agendas, alternatives and public policies. Boston: Little Brown & Co

Kingdon, J.W. (1995). Agendas, Alternatives, and Public Policies. 2nd edn. New York: HarperCollins

Kirkpatrick, C and Mosedale, S. (2001). European governance report: the role of sustainability impact assessment. Institute for Development Policy and Management. Manchester, UK: University of Manchester

Kirkpatrick, C.,Lee, N and Morrissey, O.(1999). WTO new round: sustainability impact assessment study. Phase one report. Institute for Development Policy and Management. Manchester, UK: University of Manchester

Kremer, M and Edward, M. (2007). The illusion of sustainability. Quarterly Journal of Economics 122 3): 1007–65.

LaFond, A and Brown, L. (2003). A guide to monitoring and evaluation of capacity-building interventions in the health sector in developing countries. Measure Evaluation Manual Series, No. 7. Carolina Population Center, University of North Carolina at Chapel Hill. 2003

LaFond, A.K., Brown, L and Macintyre, K. (2002). Mapping capacity in the health sector: a conceptual framework. Int J Health Plann Manage 2002; 17 (1):3-22.

LaPelle, N., Zapka, J and Ockene, J.K (2006). Sustainability of public health programmes: the example of tabacco treatment services in Massachusetts. Am. J Public Health 2006 August 96 (8):1363-1369.

Langer, M.E., Schon, E., Egger-Steiner, A.M et al. (2002). Sustainable development and the evaluation process at the regional/local level. S.D.-EVA-Pro. Final report. Vienna: Abteilung fur Wirtschaft and Umwelt. Evaluation of sustainable development.

Levine, R., Rosenmoller, M and Khaleghian, P. (2001). Financial Sustainability of Childhood Immunisation: Issues and options. Global Alliance for Vaccines and Immunisations. Available at http://www, vaccinealliance.org/financing/identity.htn .

Leavell, H. R., & Clark, E. G. (1979). The science and art of preventing disease, prolonging life, and promoting physical and mental health and efficiency. In Preventive Medicine for the Doctor in his Community (3rd ed.). Huntington, NY: Robert E. Krieger Publishing Company.

Lincoln, C., Evans, D., Evans, T., Sadana, R., Stilwell, B.,Travis, P.,Van Lerberghe, W and Zurn, P. (2006). World Health Report 2006: working together for health. Geneva: WHO. OCLC 71199185

Litt, J., Reed, H., Zieff, S.G.,Tabak, R.G., Eyler, A.A., Tompkins, N.O., Lyn, R., Gustat, J., Goins, K.V and Bornstein, D. (2013). Advancing environmental and policy change through active living collaboratives: compositional and stakeholder engagement correlates of group effectiveness. J Public Health

Management Practice, 2013, 19(3) E-Supp, S49–S57

Maeda, A., Harrit, M.N., Mabuchi, S., Siadat, B and Nagpal, S. ().Creating evidence for better health financing decisions: a strategic guide for the institutionalization of national health accounts. Amazon. Com. Available at https://www.amazon.com/Creating-Evidence-Better-Financing-Decisions/dp/B01F9R728Q

Marjan VanHerwijnen. (2008). Chapter 4, the sustainability A-test. Institute for Environmental Studies, VU University, Amsterdam. Available at hppp://asset.keep eek.cache.com/medias/domain21/-pdf/media1012/164008-hnoek2vjbs/large/2.jpg

Markwell, S. (2010). Identifying and managing internal and external stakeholder interests. Available at http://www.healthknowledge.org.uk/public-health-textbook/organisation-management/5b-understanding-ofs/managing-internal-external-stakeholders

MacFarlane, S., Racelis, M and Muli-Musiime, F. (2000). Public health in developing countries. Lancet 356 (2000): 841-846

Manning, G., Kent, C and McMillen, S. (1996). Building community: the human side of work. Cincinnati, Ohio: Thomson Executives Press.

Mays, GP., Smith, SA., Ingram, RC., Racster, LR., Lamberth, C.D and Lovely, C.S. (2009). Public health delivery systems: evidence, uncertainty and emergency research Needs. American Journal of Preventive Medicine. Available at www.rwjf.org/en/research-publications/find-rwjf-research.html?pr=Elservier.

Medical Library Association. (2004). Evidence-based public health: finding and appraising relevant resources. Medical Library Continuing Education Course. Available at http://library.umassmed.edu/obpph/characteristic.ppt

Meister, J.S and Guernsey de Zapien, J. (2005). Bringing health policy issues front and center in the community: expanding the role of community health coalitions. Prev Chronic Dis. Available at URL: http://www.cdc.gov/pcd/issues/2005/jan/04_0080.htm.

Merson, M.H., Black, R.E & Mills, A.J. (2006). International public health: diseases, programmes, systems, and policies. Jones and Baretlett Publishing, Inc.

Melgaard, B., Creese, A., Aylward, B., Oliver, J.M., Maher, C et al. (1998). Disease eradication and health systems development. In: Goodman RA et al., eds.Global disease elimination and eradication as public health strategies. Proceedings of a conference held in Atlanta, Georgia, USA, 23±25 February 1998. Bulletin of the World Health Organization, 1998,75 (Suppl. 2): 26±31.

McKenzie, J., Pinger, R and Kotechi, J.E .(2011). An introduction to community health. Canada: Jones and Bartlett Publishers

Ministry of Health & Social Welfare. (2001). Gambia EPI Review. Banjul: MOH&SW

Ministry of Health & Social Welfare (2013). National health accounts. A briefing of the NHA national steering committee, The Quadrangle. Banjul. MOH&SW,

Ministry of Health & Social Welfare. (2003). Financial sustainability plan. MOH&SW.

Ministry of Health & Social Welfare. (2001). Review of the programme of immunisation. MOH&SW

Ministry of Finance and Economic Affairs. (2005). Estimates of revenue and expenditure 2005. Banjul: MOF&EA

Mills, A., Palmer, N., Gilson, L., McIntyre, S., Sinnanovic, E and Wadee, H. (2004). Improving the quality of primary health care: public and private provision. ID21 Research Highlights, 25 November.

Mokdad, A. H., Marks, J. S., Stroup, D. F and Gerberding, J. L. (2004). Actual causes of death in the United States, 2000. Journal of the American Medical Association,291(10), 1238-1245.

Nachega, J.B., Kthman, A.O., Ho, Y.S., Lo, M., Anude, C., Kayembe, P et al. (2012). Current status and future prospects of epidemiology and public health training and research in the WHO African Region. Int. J Epidemiol 2012, Dec

41(6): 1829-46.dol:10.1093/ije/dys 189

National Academy of Sciences. (2011). Improving health in the United States: the role of health impact assessment. Available at http:// www.acbi.nlon.nih.gov/books/NBK83548.

National Network of Public Health Institute. (2010).Programmes. Available at nnphi.org/program-areas/accreditation-ad-performance-improvement/ programs

National Network of Public Health Institutes. (2010). Community of practice for public health improvement (COPPHI). Available at http://nnphi.org/ program-areas/acccreditation and performance-improvement/programs of nursing science.com

Olafsdottir, A.E., Pokhrel, S., Allotey, P and Reidpath, D.D. (2012). The fallacy of the equity-efficiency trade-of: re-thinking the efficient health care system. BMC Public Health 2012, 12 (suppl 1):53 Doi 10. 1186/1471-2458-12-51 -53

Organisation for Economic Co-operation and Development. (2003). OECD Health data: a comparative analysis of 30 Countries. Organisation for Economic Co-operation and Development, Centre de Recherche d'âtude et de Documentation en âconomie de la Santâ (CREDES), OECD

Organisation for Economic Cooperation and Development. (2000). The contribution of human and social capital to sustained economic growth and well-being. Canada: OECD

Organisation for Economic Cooperation and Development. (2011).Where is the money and what are we doing with it?: a strategic guide for the institutionalisation of national health accounts. Available at www.oecd.org/els/health systems/48852492.pdf

Organisation for Economic Cooperation and Development. (2010). Guidance on sustainability impact assessment. Available at www.oecd.org/ greengrowth/46530443.pdf

Oxford University. (1982). Oxford English Dictionary. Oxford University Press

Partnership for Health Reform. (2003). Understanding national health accounts: the methodology and implementation process. Bethesda, MD: PHR Project

Rannan-Eliya,R. P., Nada, K.H., Kamal, A.M and Ali, A.I. (1994). Egypt's national health accounts 1994-1995.Special Initiatives Report No. 3. Bethesda, Maryland, USA: Partnerships for Health Reform, Abt Associates Inc

Rannan-Eliya, R.P and Berman, P. (1994). National health accounts in developing countries: improving the foundation. Boston, Massachusetts: Data for Decision Making, Department of Population and International Health, Harvard School of Public Health

Reidpath, D.D; Olafsdottir, A.E; Pokhrel, S & Allotey, P (2012). The fallacy of the equity-efficiency trade-off: rethinking the efficient health system. BMC Public Health 2012, 12 (supp. l): 53 doi 10.1186/1471-2458-12-51-53
Rannan-Eli
Ruderman, M (2000). Resource guide to concepts and methods for community -based and collaborative problem-solving, Women's and Children's Health Policy Centre, Department of Population and Family Health Sciences, John Hopkins University School of Public Health. Available at http:// www.jhsph.edu/research centre-and-institutes
Richardson, J.T.E. (1997. Handbook of qualitative research methods for psychology and social sciences. Leicester, UK: The British Psychological Society books, Biddles LTD.
Robertson, R., Davies, J and Jobe, K. (1984).Service volume and other factors affecting the costs of immunizations in the Gambia. Bulletin of the World Health Organization,62(5):729.736(1984)
Rovniak, L.S., Hovell, M.F., Wojcik, J.R., Winett, R.A., Martinez-Donate, A.P. (2005). Enhancing theoretical fidelity: an e-mail-based walking programme demonstration. Am J Health Promot. 2005;20(2):85–95.
Rogers, E.M. (2003). Diffusion of Innovations. 5th ed New York, NY: Free Press
Rychetnik, L., Frommer, M., Hawe, P and A Shiell. (2002). Criteria for evaluating evidence on public health interventions. Epidemiol Community Health 2002;56:119-127 doi:10.1136/jech.56.2.119

Sachs, J.D and McArthur, J. (2005). The milleniunproject: a plan for meeting the millennium development goals. Lancet, 365,347-353
Sarr, F. (2005). Assessing the sustainability of the expansion of the expanded programme on Immunisation inThe Gambia. PhD thesis. London: London South Bank University, UK
Sarriot, E.G., Winch, P.J., Ryan, L.J., Bowie, J., Kouletio, M., Swedberg, E., LeBan, K., Edison, J., Welch, R and Pacqué, M.C. (2004).A methodological approach and framework for sustainability assessment in NGO-implemented primary health care programmes. Int J Health Plann Manage. 2004 Jan-Mar;19 (1):23-41.
Sabatier, P. A. (1993) Policy change over a decade or more. In Sabatier, P. A. and Jenkins-Smith, H. C. (eds) Policy Change and Learning: An Advocacy

Coalition Approach. Westview Press, Boulder, C

Streefland P., Harnmeijer, JW and Chabot J.(1995). Implications of economic crisis and structural ad-justment policies for PHC in the periphery. In: Chabot J, Harnmeijer JW, Streefland P, editors.African primary health care in times of economic turbulence. Amsterdam: KIT Press; 1995. p. 11–9

Steadman, H.J., Cocozza, JJ., Dennis, D.L, et al. Successful programme maintenance when federal demonstration dollars stop: the ACCEhSS programme for homeless mentally ill persons. Adm Policy Ment Health. 2002;29 (6):481–493.

Shearer, J.C., Walker, D.G., Risko, N and Levine, O.S. (2012). The impact of new vaccine introduction on the coverage of existing vaccines: a cross-national, multivariable analysis.. Vaccine. 2012 Dec 14; 30(52):7582-7. Epub 2012 Oct 23

Scott, J and Marshall, G .(2009). Operational definition (operationalisation). A Dictionary of Sociology (3 rev.ed). Available at http://oxfordindex.oup.com/view/10.1093/acref/9780199533008.013.1615

Schiller, C;. Winters, M., Hanson, H.M and Ashe, M.C .(2013). A framework for stakeholder identification in concept mapping and health research: a novel process and its application older adult mobility and the built environment. BMC Public health 2013, 13: 428 doi: 10.1186/1471-2458-13-428

Schell, S.F., Luke, AD., Schooley. M.W., Elliott, M.B., Harper, S.H., Muller, N.B and Bunger, A.C. (2013). Public health programme capacity for sustainability: a new framework. Implementation Science 2013, 8;15 doi: 101186/1748-5908-8-15

Scheirer, MA. (1990).The life cycle of an innovation: adoption versus discontinuation of the fluoride mouth rinse programme in schools. J Health Soc Behav. 1990;31(2):203–215

Scheirer, M.A., Hartling, G., Hagerman .D. (2008). Defining sustainability outcomes of health programmes: illustrations from an online survey. Eval Program Plann. 2008;31(4):335–346

Schmeer, K. (1999). Guidelines for conducting a stakeholder analysis. Bethesda MD: Partnerships for Health Reform Projects

Scott Peck, M.(1993). Chapter III The true meaning of community in the different drum: community making and peace. Available at http://www.entcom.eu/wp-content/uploads/2015/10/Entcom-WS-Report-Annex2.pdf

Smith, D., Peterson, W.E., Jaglarz, M., Doell, K., Dearing, J.W and, Kreuter, M.W. (2010) Designing for diffusion of cancer communication innovations. Patient Educ Couns. 2010;81(suppl 1):S100–S110

Smith, S., Peterson, W.E., Jaglarz, M and Doell, K. (2009). Improving access to preventive services for marginalized families during early childhood: an integrative review of inter-organizational integration interventions.The Open Health Services and Policy Journal , 2009, 2: 16-25

Srinivas, H. (2015).The seven triads of sustainability. Available at http://www.gdrc.org/sustdev/triads/triad7.html

Stirman, S. W., Kimberly, J., Cook, N., Calloway,A., Castro, F and Charns, M. (2012).The sustainability of new programmes and innovations: a review of the empirical literature and recommendations for future research. Implement Sci. 2012; 7: 17.

Swerissen, H and Crisp, B.R. (2004). The sustainability of health promotion interventions for different levels of social organizations. Health Promot Int 2004;19:123–30

The Association of Faculties of Medicine of Canada. (2007).Theory thinking about health, chapter 4, basic concepts in prevention surveillance and health promotion, the stages of prevention. AFMC Primer on Population Health. Available at http://phprimer.afmc.ca/Part1-

The University of Sydney (2012) What is policy?. Available at http://sydney.edu.au/legal/policy/what/index.shtml

The Institute of Health Systems. (20909). National health accounts: training manual for implementing national health asccounts in India. The Institute of Health Systems, HACA Bhavan, Hyderabad, India. Available at www.ihsnet.org.in/publication/NHA Manual.pdf=page=287zoom=auto-23,=s4 .

Toman, M A., Lile, R and King, D.(1998). Assessing sustainability: some conceptual and empirical challenges. Available at http://www.rff.org/files/sharepoint/WorkImages/Download/RFF-DP-98-42.pdf

University of Pittsburgh. (2014). Concept mapping overview. Concept Mapping Institute. Available at public health.pitt.edu/behavior al-and-community-health-sciences.

University of Manchester. (2014). Public health & occupational health. Manchester: University of Manchester Centre for the History of Science Technology

United Nations .(1992). United nations conference on the environment and development. New York: UN

United Nations Development Programme. (2004). Human development report. Available at http:///www.hdr.undp.org/en/content/human-development-report-2004

United Nations General Assembly. (2015). Draft outcome document of the United Nations summit for the adoption of the post-2015 development agenda.

New York: UN.

United Nations. (2006). The millennium development goals: what are they?. Available at www.unmilleniumprojectUNDP, New York

United Nations (2015). Sustainable development goals. Available at www.un.org/sustainable development/sustainable- development-goals

US Department of State. (2009).The Bretton Woods conference, 1944. Available at
https://2001-2009.state.gov/r/pa/ho/time/wwii/98681.htm

United States General Accounting Office. (1999). Factors contributing to low vaccination rates in developing countries. Report to Congressional Requesters. Washington: USGAO.

Van Herwijnen, M. (2008). SustainabilityA-Test. OECD. Available at www.oecd.org/greengrowth/39924800.pdf

Varvasovszky, Z and McKee, M. 1998. An analysis of alcohol policy in Hungary: who is in charge? Addiction 93(12): 1815–27

Waddington, C. (2004).Does earmarked donor funding make it more or less likely that developing countries will allocate their resources towards programmes that yield the greatest health benefits?. Bulletin of the World Health Organization 2004;82:703-708.

Walt, G. (1994). Health policy. London: Zed Books

Weiss, CH. (1997).Theory-based evaluation: why aren't we doing it?. New Dir Program Eval. 1997;76:41–55

Williams, A. (2008). The enemies of progress, Vol 34, Societas; Essays in Political and Cultural Criticism.

Winstanley, D., Sorabji, D and Dawson, S.(1995).When the pieces don't fit: a stakeholder power matrix to analyse public sector restructuring. Public Money & Management, p. 19-26. apr/june 1995

Wise Geek (2003). What are the different types of sustainability issues. Available athttp://www.wisegeek.com/what-are-the-differeny-types-of-sustainability issues.htm

World Bank. (1993). World development report: investing in health. 1-350. 1993.

World Commission on the Environment and Development. (1987). Brundtland report. New York: WCED

World Health Organisation. (1946). Frequently asked questions from the "Preamble to the Constitution of the World Health Organization" as adopted by the International Health Conference, 1946

World Health Organisation. (2001). Macro-economic and health: investing in

health for economic development. Geneva: WHO.
World Health Organisation. (2003). WHO definition of health. Available at http://www.who.int/about/definition/en/print.html
World Health Organization. (2014). The top 10 causes of death. The Open Health Services and Policy Journal,2009,2,16-25 (n.d.). Available at: http://www.who.int/mediacentre/factsheets/fs310/en/index2.html
World Health Organisation.(2008). Closing the gap- WHO report on social determinants of health. Geneva: WHO Commission on Social Determinants of Health. Available at http://whqlibdoc.who.int/publications/2008/9789241563703_eng.pdf?ua=1
World Health Organisation. (2014). The world health report 2008- primary health care -now more than ever. Geneva: WHO.
World Health Organization. (1978). Primary health care. Geneva: WHO.
World Health Organisation. (1998). The world health report 1998 – Life in the 21st century: a vision for al. Geneva: WHO.
World Health Organization. (2011) Health policy. Geneva: WHO.
World Health Organisation/Pan-American Health Organisation. (2000-2007). Essential public health functions as a strategy for improving health systems performance: trends and challenges
since the Public Health in the Americas Initiatives 2000-2007. Available at www.nwph.net/hawa/writed/1560who Pan American Health Organisation.pdf.
World Health Organisation. (2015). The top 10 causes of death. Available at www.who.int/media centre/factsheets/fs310/en/index2-html.
World Health Organisation. (2015). Public health. Available at www.who.int/trade/glossary/story o76/en/
World Health Organisation. (2001). Health impact assessment in development policy and planning: report of an informal WHO consultative meeting, Cartagena,Colombia.
World Health Organisation. (2000). The world health report 2000: Health system-improving performance. 1-206. Geneva: WHO, 85(7):511-8.
World Health Organisation. (2002). The common assessment tool for immunization services. Geneva: WHO
World Health Organization. (1986). Ottawa charter on health promotion. Geneva: WHO.
World Health Organisation. (2012). Vaccination in humanitarian emergencies: iterature review and case studies. Available at http://www.who.int/immunization/sage/meetings/2012/
april/2_SAGE_WGVHE_SG1__Lit_Review_CaseStudies.pdf
Widdus, R. (1999). Adoption of new vaccines. Keynote address to the South Pacific Immunisation Conference. Brisbone, Australia

Yin RK, Heald KA, Vogel ME. (1977).Tinkering with the system. Lexington, MA: Lexington Books.

Index

Printed in the United States
By Bookmasters